Step b

CT S

Step by Step

CT Scan

(A Practical Guide for Residents and Technologists)

D Karthikeyan DMRD DNB
Chief Radiologist
Division of Computed Tomography and Body Imaging
Department of Imaging Sciences
KG Hospital and Postgraduate Institute
Coimbatore
Programme Director, Radeducation Pvt. Ltd.
Coimbatore

Deepa Chegu
Consultant Radiologist
GEM Hospital (P) Ltd
Coimbatore

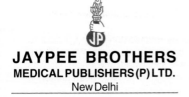

JAYPEE BROTHERS
MEDICAL PUBLISHERS (P) LTD.
New Delhi

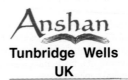

Tunbridge Wells
UK

First published in the UK by

Anshan Ltd
in 2006
6 Newlands Road
Tunbridge Wells
Kent TN4 9AT, UK

Tel/Fax: +44 (0)1892 557767
E-mail: info@anshan.co.uk
www.anshan.co.uk

ISBN-10 1 904798 810
ISBN-13 978 1 904798 81 1

British Library Cataloguing in Publication Data
A catalogue record for this book is available from the British Library

Printed in India by Paras Offset Pvt. Ltd., Naraina, New Delhi.

Preface

Since the introduction of computed tomography in the 70's, there has been tremendous changes in the way CT is performed resulting in a broad positive impact on patient management. This book has been designed as a primer which gives a practical insight into the principles and practice of computed tomography for radiology residents and technicians.

D Karthikeyan
Deepa Chegu

Contents

Contents

Chapter 1

History and Basics

GN Hounsfield, a senior research scientist in Middlesex, England announced the invention of a revolutionary imaging technique. In the year 1972, that he called computed axial transverse scanning (*tomos*—meaning section, *graphy*—picture in Greek).

He presented a cross-sectional image of the head that revealed the internal structures of the brain in a manner previously only seen at surgery or autopsy and for the first time pathologic processes such as blood clots, tumors, and strokes could be easily seen non-invasively.

COMMON NAMES

a. Computerized axial transverse scanning (Hounsfield, 1972)
b. Computerized axial tomography (CAT)
c. X-ray computed tomography (X-ray CT)
d. Computed/computerized tomography (CT)

Computed tomography (CT) is currently the preferred name.

HISTORY LEADING TO CT SCAN

- 1917—Radon developed the basic mathematical equations.
- 1940—Frank and Takahashi published the basic principles of axial CT.
- 1956—Cormack developed theory of image reconstruction.
- 1967—Hounsfield developed the clinically useful CT scanner.
- 1973—First clinical brain scanner in Mayo Clinic.

Hounsfield and Cormack shared the 1979 Nobel Prize for their development of CT.

CONVENTIONAL TOMOGRAPHY (Fig. 1.1)

Conventional radiographs provide an integrated, 2D view of a 3D distribution of a object μ (x, y, z) with superimposition of all structures. The disadvantage of this method is:

1. Depth information is lost.
2. Overlapping structures may interfere with diagnosis, and subtle differences in contrast is lost.
3. Not quantitative.

Tomo (="cut or section") + graph (="something written or drawn") = tomograph.

X-ray tomography an analog technique suggested in 1914 by Mayer, Bocage, Grossman, and Vallebona all developed the idea further and built their own equipment.

Method

a. X-ray source on one side of subject and film on another, diagonally opposed.
b. Source and detector move at constant rates in opposite directions.
c. Source and detector distances from the imaging plane and rate of motion determined such that objects in the imaging plane always project to the same relative locations on the film.
d. Objects out of the plane project to several locations and are thus blurred.

Three basic goals of computed tomography were based to rectify the pitfalls of conventional tomography, they are:
- To overcome superimposition of structures.
- To improve the contrast of the image.
- To measure small differences in tissue contrast.
  These three goals were accomplished by:
- Transmitting a collimated X-ray beam through a specific cross-section of the body.
- Detectors that can measure small differences in tissue contrast.
- A computer that allows data to be manipulated and enhanced.

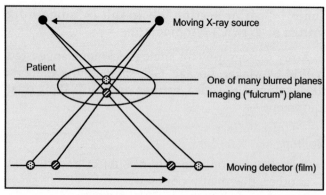

Fig. 1.1: Conventional tomography

INTRODUCTION—EQUIPMENT

The basic principle behind CT is that the internal structure of an object can be reconstructed from multiple projections of the object. The patient lies on the table within the CT gantry, which is shaped like a giant donut. During each slice acquisition, an X-ray tube circling the patient produces an X-ray beam that passes through the patient and is absorbed by a ring of detectors surrounding the patient (Fig. 1.2). The intensity of the X-ray beam that reaches the detectors is dependent on the absorption characteristics of the tissues it passes through. Since the beam is moving around the patient, each tissue will be exposed from multiple directions. Using a process called Fourier analysis, the computer uses the information obtained from the different amounts of X-ray absorption to reconstruct the density and position of the different structures contained within each slice.

A thin cross-section of the human body, or a tomographic slice, can be reconstructed from images, or projections, taken from multiple angles around the human body.

CT images show a radiographic difference in the various soft tissues and structures forming the human body. Projections are obtained by passing an X-ray beam through the object at different angles and measuring the transmitted radiation.

Then, the internal structure of an object can be reconstructed by adding multiple projections of the object: X-rays passing through a body section are attenuated at different rates by different tissues (Figs 1.3 and 1.4).

System Components of CT Scanner

Three main components are—gantry assembly, computer, operating console.

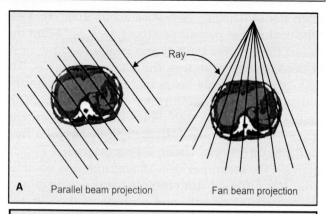

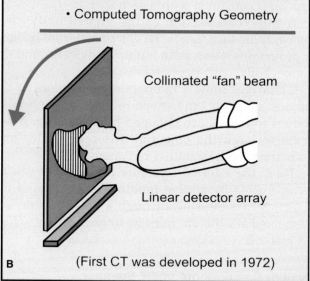

Figs 1.2A and B: Tomographic images are produced from a large number of X-ray transmission measurements called rays, a group of rays acquired in a certain geometry is called a projection or view. Two different geometries are used in CT, parallel beam and fan beam projection

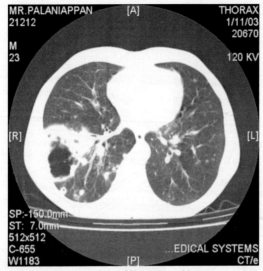

Fig. 1.3: Axial CT section of lungs

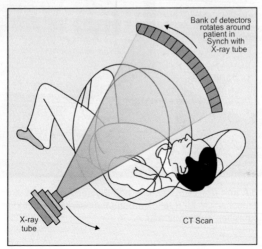

Fig. 1.4: Schematic diagram depicting tube rotation

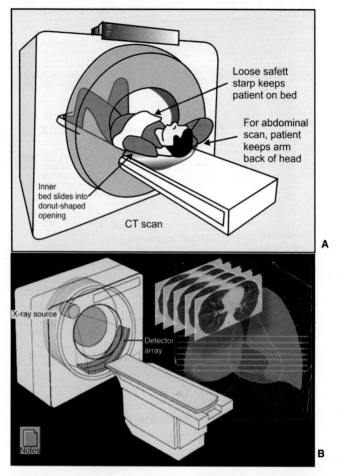

Figs 1.5A and B: The X-ray tube and the detector or set of detectors, and the mechanism for rotation around the patient are included into the data acquisition system (DAS)

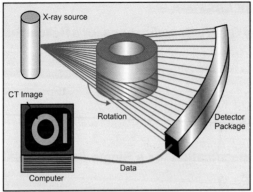

Fig. 1.6: Schematic diagram showing the data acquisition system (DAS)

Hardware Consideration

A. X-ray tube
B. Collimators
C. Detectors—Scintillation crystals
   Xenon gas ionisation chambers.

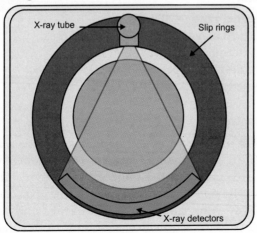

Fig. 1.7: Schematic diagram showing the CT scan gantry assembly

GANTRY ASSEMBLY

General Gantry Specifications for a Helical Scanner

- Aperture—65 cm.
- Tilt— +/- 20 degree.
- Tiltspeed—1 degree/second.
- Height to isocetre—90 cm.
- Rotation speed—360° in 1.5, 2, 3, 5 seconds.

Tube Specification for a Single Slice Helical Scanner

- Anode heat capacity—2 to 3.5 MHU.
- Anode heat deception—500 khu/min.
- Casing heat deception—275 khu/min.
- Focal size—0.7 mm × 0.6 mm.

Table Specification for a Single Slice Helical Scanner

- Vertical range—40 to 90 cm.
- Vertical elevation speed—17 mm/sec.
- Maximum cradle travel—152 cm.
- Cradle travel speed—20 to 100 mm/sec.
- Table load capacity—205 kg.

CT Gantry

The first major component of a CT system is referred to as the scan or imaging system. The imaging system primarily includes the gantry and patient table or couch. The gantry is a moveable frame that contains the X-ray tube including collimators and filters, detectors, data acquisition system (DAS), rotational components including slip ring systems and all associated electronics such as gantry angulation motors and positioning laser lights.

In older CT systems a small generator supplied power to the X-ray tube and the rotational components via cables for operation. This type of generator was mounted on the rotational component of the CT system and rotated with the X-ray tube. Some generators remain mounted inside the gantry wall.

Some newer scanner designs utilize a generator that is located outside the gantry. Slip ring technology eliminated the need for cables and allows continuous rotation of the gantry components. The inclusion of slip ring technology into a CT system allows for continuous scanning without interference of cables. A CT gantry can be angled up to 30° toward a forward or backward position. Gantry angulation is determined by the manufacturer and varies among CT systems. Gantry angulation allows the operator to align pertinent anatomy with the scanning plane. The opening through which a patient passes is referred to as the gantry aperture.

Gantry aperture diameters generally range from 50 to 85 cm. Generally, larger gantry aperture diameters, 70 to 85 cm, are necessary for CT departments that do a large volume of biopsy procedures. The larger gantry aperture allows for easier manipulation of biopsy equipment and reduces the risk of injury when scanning the patient and the placement of the biopsy needle simultaneously. The diameter of the gantry aperture is different for the diameter of the scanning circle or scan field of view. If a CT system has a gantry aperture of 70 cm diameter it does not mean that you can acquire patient data utilizing a 70 cm diameter.

Generally, the scanning diameter in which patient or projection data is acquired is less than the size of the gantry aperture. Lasers or high intensity lights are included within or mounted on the gantry. The lasers or high intensity lights serve as anatomical positioning guides that reference the center of the axial, coronal, and sagittal planes.

X-RAY TUBE, COLLIMATION, FILTRATION

X-ray Sources

X-ray is produced by an X-ray tube. The three main parts of any X-ray tube are the anode, cathode and the filament. When the filament is heated, electrons are ejected from its surface. A large voltage between the cathode and the anode force electrons to accelerate towards the anode. The electrons hitting the anode (tungsten) produce Bremstrahlung radiation at an efficiency of only 1 percent. The other 99 percent of the electrons energy is converted into heat.

> Most modern system use tubes with two focal spots small spot is used for high resolution examination. And large spot is used for larger anatomic coverage.

Stationary anode—Used in eary scanners, oil cooled, large focal spot giving rise to higher potential radiation.

Rotating anode—Aircooled, small focal spot requires large heat capacity and fast cooling rates.

Mechanical stresses due to tube rotation—Up to 13 G for 0.5 second rotation.

CT procedures facilitate the use of large exposure factors, (high mA and kVp values) and short exposure

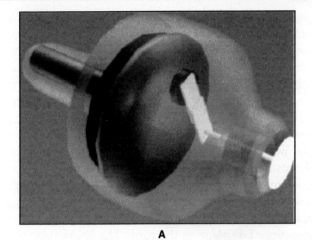

A

B

Figs 1.8A and B: (A) Rotating anode; (B) Conventional tube

times. The development of spiral/helical CT allows continuous scanning while the patient table or couch moves through the gantry aperture. A typical spiral/helical CT scan of the abdomen may require the continuous production of X-rays for a 30 to 40 second period. The stress caused by the constant build up of heat can lead to a rapid decrease of tube life. When an X-ray tube reaches a maximum heat value it simply will not operate until it cools down to an acceptable level. CT systems produce X-radiation continuously or in short millisecond bursts or pulses at high mA and kVp values. CT X-ray tubes must possess a high heat capacity which is the amount of heat that a tube can store without operational damage to the tube. The X-ray tube must be designed to absorb high heat levels generated from the high speed rotation of the anode and the bombardment of electrons upon the anode surface.

An X-ray tubes heat capacity is expressed in heat units. Modern CT systems utilize X-ray tubes that have a heat capacity of approximately 3.5 to 5 million heat unit (MHU). A CT X-ray tube must possess a high heat dissipation rate. Many CT X-ray tubes utilize a combination of oil and air cooling systems to eliminate heat and maintain continuous operational capabilities.

A CT X-ray tube anode has a large diameter with a graphite backing. The large diameter backed with graphite allows the anode to absorb and dissipate large amounts of heat. The focal spot size of an X-ray tube is determined by the size of the filament and cathode which is determined by the manufacturer. Most X-ray tubes have more than one focal spot size. The use of a small focal spot increases detail but it concentrates heat onto a smaller portion of the anode, therefore, more heat is generated. As previously described, when heat is building up faster than the tube can dissipate it the X-ray tube will not produce X-rays until it has sufficiently cooled. CT tubes utilize a bigger filament than conventional radiography X-ray tubes. The use of a bigger filament increases the size of the effective focal spot.

Decreasing the anode or target angle decreases the size of the effective focal spot. Generally, the anode angle of a conventional radiography tube is between 12 and 17 degrees. CT tubes employ a target angle approximately between 7 and 10 degrees. The decreased anode or target angle also helps aleviate some of the effects caused by the heel effect.

CT can compensate any loss of resolution due the use of larger focal spot sizes by employing resolution enhancement algorithms such as bone or sharp algorithms, targeting techniques, and decreasing section thickness.

Collimation

Important Component for Reducing Patient Dose and Improving Image Quality by Reducing Scatter Radiation

In CT collimation of the X-ray beam includes tube collimators, a set of pre-patient collimators and post-patient or pre-detector collimators. Some CT systems utilize this type of collimation system while other do not. The tube or source collimators are located in the X-ray tube and determine the section thickness that will be utilized for a particular CT scanning procedure. When the CT technologist selects a section thickness he or she is determining tube collimation by narrowing or widening the beam.

A second set of collimators located directly below the tube collimators maintain the width of the beam as it travels toward the patient. A final set of collimators called post-patient or pre-detector collimators are located below the patient and above the detector. The primary responsibilities of this set of collimators are to insure proper beam width at the detector and reduce the number of scattered photons that may enter a detector.

Pre-patient collimation
- Depends on the focal spot size
- Mounted on the tube housing
- Creates more parallel beam
- Reduces patient dose

Pre-detector collimation
- Restricts the field of view of detectors
- Reduces the scatter radiation on the detector
- Aperture width helps determine the slice thickness

The X-ray field is filtered to reduce the low energy X-rays which are not useful for imaging but that increase the radiation dose received by the patient. This process is called collimation.

The beam undergoes two-levels of collimation: (1) source collimation, and (2) detector collimation.

The source collimator controls the thickness of the tomographic slice (most common thickness are 1, 2, 5 or 10 mm).

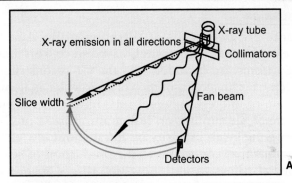

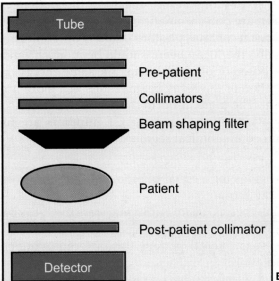

Figs 1.9A and B: Schematic diagram showing the relationship between detectors and collimators

Filtration

There are two types of filtration utilized in CT. Mathematical filters such as bone or soft tissue algorithms are included into the CT reconstruction process to enhance resolution of a particular anatomical region of interest. Inherent tube filtration and filters made of aluminium or Teflon are utilized in CT to shape the beam intensity by filtering out low energy photons that contribute to the production of scatter. Special filters called "bow-tie" filters absorb low energy photons before reaching the patient. X-ray beams are polychromatic in nature which means an X-ray beam contains photons of many different energies. Ideally, the X-ray beam should be monochromatic or composed of photons having the same energy. Heavy filtration of the X-ray beam results in a more uniform beam. The more uniform the beam, the more accurate the attenuation values or CT numbers are for the scanned anatomical region.

Provides for a equal photon distribution across the X-ray beam.

Allows equal beam hardening were the X-ray passes through the filter and object.

Lessens overall patient dose by removing softer radiation.

Made of aluminium, grafite can be curved, wedge or flat in shape.

Detectors

Detectors gather information by measuring the X-ray attenuation through objects.

The most important properties of X-ray detectors used in CT are:

a. Efficiency
b. Response time (after glow)
c. Linearity

Efficiency is related to the number of X-rays reaching the detector that are detected.

Response time is related to how fast the detected X-ray is converted into an electrical pulse or current.

Linearity is related to the proportionality between the output of the detector and the number of incident X-rays.

The two types of detector that have been used for CT are:

- *Scintillation detectors:* Use solid materials in which the energy of X-rays is converted to light photons. Then, the emitted light is converted into an electrical current by using a photomultiplier tube or a silicon photodiode. The material which produces light when the X-ray energy is absorbed is named scintillator and the combination of a scintillator and the device converting light into a current, is named scintillation detector.

- *Gas ionization detectors:* These are based on the ionization of a gas inside a closed chamber when the X-ray energy is absorbed into a gas. The main disadvantage is the low efficiency of gas detectors.

Favourable Detector Characters

- High absorption efficiency.
- High conversion efficiency.
- High capture efficiency.
- High reproducibility and stability.

Scintillation Detectors

- Uses a scintillation crystal coupled to a photo-multiplier tube to convert light to electrons.
- Amount of light produced is proportional to the energy of the absorbed X-rays.
- Used in older generation of machines.
- Disadvantage is that of after glow.

Examples—Sodium iodide, cadmium tungstate, caesium iodide.

Gas Detectors

- Ionization chamber that uses xenon or krypton gas.
- Ionized gas causes electrons to attach to tungsten plates creating electronic signals.
- Gas that is ionized is proportional to the incident radiation.
- 100% effective utilization of energy.

  Ionization chamber—xenon (underpressure).

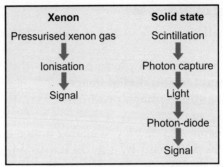

Fig. 1.10: Schematic diagram showing the
mechanism of xenon and solid state detector

Operator Console

Scan Console

- Technical factors, slice thickness, no of scans, angle of gantry.
- Initiates scan, record patient data, sets FOV.

Display Console

- Used to manipulate post scan data,
- Post processing work—measurements, MIPS, 3D formations.
- Window level and width.

Computer

The computer processes convert the signal from analog to digital by using a analog to digital convertor. It stores the digital signal during the scan and reconstructs the images after the scan is complete. This reconstruction can be done immediately or later. Data can be manipulated to reconstruct into various planes.

Summary of Processes

The formation of a CT image is a distinct three phase process.

- The reconstruction phase processes the acquired data and forms a digital image.
- The scanning phase produces data, but not an image.
- The visible and displayed analog image (shades of grey) is produced by the digital-to analog conversion phase.

X-ray CT system

- Thinly collimated X-ray beam
- Multiple views
- Detectors to collect X-ray photons
- Data acquisition system
- Image reconstruction algroithm (filtered back projection)
- Film/monitors to display axial slices

Fig. 1.11: Summary of CT image formation

IMAGE RECONSTRUCTION

The computer receives a signal in analog form and converts it to a binary digit by using a analog to digital convertor. The digital signal is stored and the image is reconstructed after the scan is over.

Each picture is displayed on a matrix, each square in a matrix is called a pixel, its assigned a number based on the amount of energy reaching the detector. This number is called as Hounsfield unit.

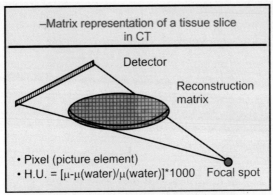

–Matrix representation of a tissue slice
in CT

Detector

Reconstruction
matrix

- Pixel (picture element)
- H.U. = [μ-μ(water)/μ(water)]*1000   Focal spot

Fig. 1.12: Schematic diagrams demonstrating the
concept of pixel and voxel

The reconstructed anatomy of an object is in the
digital format composed of a large number of Tiny
elongated blocks. Representing a volume of tissue
called voxel (Figs 1.12 and 1.13).

Voxel—3D tissue element that has a width, height
and depth. *Depth of a voxel is a important parameter which
depends on the slice thickness and each unit is assigned a
shade of grey.*

Pixel is the 2D projection of a voxel on the computer
screen and it has only height and width.

CT NUMBERS

CT Numbers and Hounsfield Units

The digital value ascribed to each pixel is called the
Hounsfield units or HU, which lies on a scale were
water has a value of 0 and air has a value of –1000.
Bone has a value in order of +1000. HU values reflect

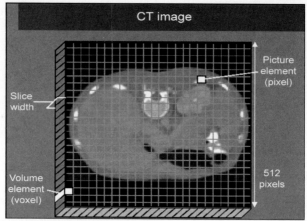

Fig. 1.13: Schematic diagram showing contents in an axial CT slice

the electron density and thus the physical composition of the voxel of tissue that the pixel represents.

Reconstruction yields linear attenuation coefficients, usually relative to that of water and scaled to a large number, the CT number.

$$CT \text{ number} = K \frac{\mu_{tissue} - \mu_{water}}{\mu_{water}}$$

Pixel values for some biological tissues are:

Tissue	CT number range in HU
Air	−1000
Lungs	−900 to −300
Fat	−120 to −80
Water	0
Muscle	10 to 30
Soft tissue	10 to 30
Cortical bone	50 to 100
Trabecular bone	500 to 1000

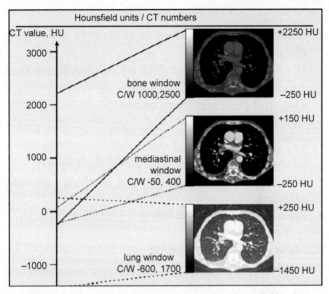

Fig. 1.14: Schematic diagram showing the Hounsfield unit

Algorithms for Image Reconstruction

The fundamental problem in CT is to calculate the linear attenuation coefficient of the pixels using a large number of X-ray transmission measurements and to use the results to build up an image of the object by means of computer processing algorithm.

An algorithm is a mathematical method for solving a problem. Various methods are used for reforming the image.

1. Back projection method
2. Iterative method
3. Analytical method.

Back Projection Method

- Simplest method also known as linear or summation method.
- Involves obtaining profiles of an object and then combining them.
- Does not produce sharp images.

Analytical Reconstruction Algorithm

- Commonly used now because of their speed.
- It is a filtered back projection method –no stair artifacts.
- Data is reconstructed using a fourier transform.

Windowing and Grey Scale

Technique of windowing is a electronic manipulation of the data to enable the shades of grey to be used to represent a limited range of HU values so that different structures can be imaged.

CT scans are displayed as a monochrome image on a TV screen. The value of the pixel at a specific point in the image is converted to a grey level. However, the range of pixel values is approximately −1000 (air) to +800 (dense bone) and the eye can only distinguish 32 grey levels at best. The majority of the soft tissues range from -100 to +100 so a system know as windowing has been developed to allow Radiologists to dynamically view images.

- Decreasing the window width increases the contrast in the image so is good for looking at differences in soft tissues.

- Increasing the window width allows structures with a large pixel range (i.e. bones and lungs) to be viewed.
- Decreasing the window level allows the lungs and other airways to be viewed.
- Increasing the window level allows the denser bones to be viewed.

Windowing allows you to dynamically alter the image. Film hard copies are taken at specific (user defined) window settings so are just a representative copy of the original image. Good diagnostic practice is to have access to the images on a diagnostic console to allow windowing to be performed as required.

Image Quality

- Spatial resolution.
- Contrast resolution.
- Noise and spatial uniformity.
- Linearity.
- Image artifacts.

Image noise and artifacts are the two biggest enemies of CT image quality. CT parameters can be manipulated to either decrease or eliminate the adverse effects of these image.

Spatial Resolution

It is the CT system's ability to differentiate small objects that are adjacent to one another. The CT scanner's resolving power relies on how well small objects that are close together but have very different attenuation values or CT numbers are imaged.

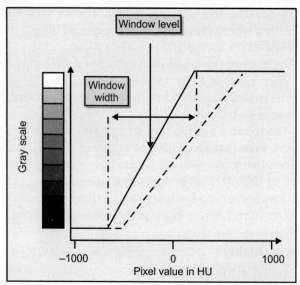

Fig. 1.15: Relationship between window level and width

There are parameters that a CT technologist can manipulate to increase the spatial resolution when scanning high frequency regions. Utilizing a bone, sharp, high frequency or high pass algorithm during reconstruction can improve the spatial resolution.

Other factors that influence spatial resolution include pixel size, which is influenced by the chosen, scanned field of view and matrix size, width of the detector, spacing between detectors, number of projections or views obtained and focal spot size.

Field of View (FOV)

• Diameter of FOV has a proved effect on the image quality.

- FOV should be adjusted to the size of the anatomic areas to be examined.
- Ideally pixels should be smaller than the minimum distance resoluble by the scanner.

Contrast Resolution

It is the ability of a CT scanner to differentiate small attenuation differences on the CT image. Contrast Resolution is also known as Low Contrast Resolution and Tissue Resolution. Contrast resolution is limited by noise, as noise in an image increases, contrast resolution decreases thereby, inhibiting the ability of the CT scanner to image slight differences in tissue density.

A soft tissue, standard or smooth algorithm is used during the reconstruction process to enhance soft tissue and contrast resolution.

Image Noise

Noise is considered to be the number one limiting factor of CT image quality. Noise is the portion of a signal that contains no information. Noise is characterized by a grainy appearance of the image.

The major types of noise include quantum noise, electronic noise and computational noise. Quantum noise is a result of too few photons reaching a detector after being attenuated by the body. Any factor that limits the number of attenuated photons at the detector will increase image noise. Anatomical structure size, reduction of slice thickness without increasing technical factors, decreasing pixel size and scatter radiation are all factors that contribute to image noise.

Electronic noise is noise contained within the image that can be caused by vibrations of any of the physical components, especially the rotational components or power fluctuations. Computational noise is primarily caused by all the statistical fluctuations that occur from the reconstruction mathematics that are essential to produce a CT image. The following factors influence image noise:

- Voxel size, slice thickness, matrix, FOV.
- Filter algorithm, mAs.

Image Artifacts

"An artifact is any distortion or error in the image that is unrelated to the subject being studied."

Artifacts can appear as geometrical inconsistencies, blurring, streaks or inaccurate CT numbers. Streak artifacts are the most common distortions or errors that affect the quality of CT images. Motion, metallic objects, out-of-field, edge gradient effects, high-low frequency interfaces, equipment malfunctions and sampling errors are all causes of streak artifacts.

Equipment malfunctions such as tube arching, electrical malfunctions and detector malfunctions produce streak artifacts on a CT image.

Source of Artifacts

- Data formation
  - Patient motion.
  - Polychromatic effects.
  - Equipment misalignment.
  - Faulty X-ray source.

CT Image Parameters—Definitions and Ranges

Noise	All CT images contain noise or pixel to pixel variations in the pixel value in the image of an object of uniform linear attenuation coefficient. It is measured as the standard deviation (σ) of the pixel values within an area of the image. The units are HU and it typically ranges from 3 to 30 HU
Spatial resolution in the image plane	This is quoted **either** as the full width at half maximum (FWHM) of the point spread function (PSF) measured in mm **or** as the spatial frequency of the 50% modulation transfer function (MTF) measured in cycles/cm. (Note percentages other than the 50% can be quoted. A simple method of converting is: $$\text{FWHM of PSF in mm} = \frac{5}{50\% \text{ of MTF in cycles/cm}}$$ The typical range of the fwhm of the PSF is from 0.75 to 2.0 mm.
Spatial resolution in the long axis	This is the slice width. The image is the "average" across the slice width so in general the spatial resolution is up to an order of magnitude poorer in this direction. This also gives rise to the partial volume effect (see later).
Dose	CT doses are measured in mGy and range upwards from about 50 mGy. CT has one of the highest dose consequences to the patient.

- Data acquisition
  - Slice geometry.
  - Profile sampling.
  - Angular sampling.

- Data measurement
  - Detector imbalance.
  - Scatter collimation.
- Data processing
  - Algorithm effects.

Because the patient moves continuously through the Gantry for a 360° rotation, the reconstructed image will be blurred with only the same filtered backprojection algorithm as conventional CT. That's why we should interpolate our image data before the filtered back-projection is used. This process leads to a higher noise level and artifacts such as stair-step artifact.

Patient Motion Artifacts (Fig. 1.16)

Motion can be voluntary or involuntary. No matter which kind of motion we are dealing with, the most efficient way to reduce motion artifact is to reduce our scanning time. Methods to reduce patient motion artifacts include patient immobilization, ECG gated CT, and some correction algorithms.

Metal Artifacts (Fig. 1.17)

Metallic materials such as prothetic devices, dental fillings, surgical clips, and electrodes produce streak artifacts on the image. Several methods have been provided to remove the artifacts coming from metal.

Beam Hardening Artifacts (Fig. 1.18)

Beam hardening is a phenomenon results from the increase of mean energy of the X-ray beam when it

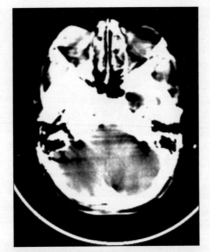

Fig. 1.16: Axial CT brain showing motion artifacts

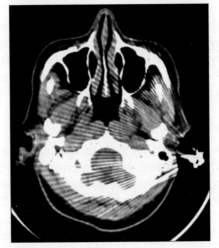

Fig. 1.17: Axial CT brain showing metal artifacts

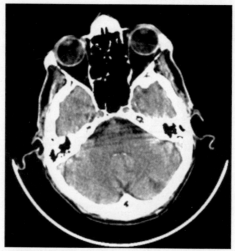

Fig. 1.18: Axial CT brain showing beam hardening artifact

passes through object. Therefore, the CT numbers of certain structures change and induce some artifacts. This kind of artifact can be reduced or eliminated with a filter that ensures the uniformity of the beam at the detectors.

Partial Volume Artifacts

Partial volume artifacts arise when a voxel contains many types of tissue. It will produce a CT number as an average of all types of tissue. This is the source of partial volume effect and will appear as bands and streaks. Using thinner slice and some computer algorithms can reduce partial volume artifacts.

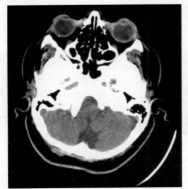

Fig. 1.19: Axial CT brain showing partial volume of clivus

Stair Step Artifacts

Apart from the well-recognized effects on the section-sensitivity profile and average image noise, the particular geometry helical CT causes complex periodic asymmetries and inconsistencies in the volumetric data sets that give rise to less-recognized effects such as variable noise distribution and section thickness.

Ring artifacts appear on a CT image as a ring or a number of rings superimposed on the structures being scanned. The artifact is commonly associated with third generation or rotate-rotate CT systems. This artifact occurs due to one or several misaligned or miscalibrated detectors in the detector array of the rotate-rotate CT system.

CT image quality is dependent upon the balancing of parameters relative to image resolution. Balancing image quality by manipulating and altering CT parameters depends upon the region or the condition being scanned with respect for patient dose. Image quality is also dependent upon limiting or eliminating the image degrading effects of noise and artifacts.

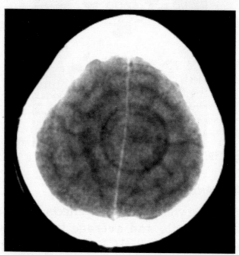

Fig. 1.20: Axial CT brain showing ring artifacts

Image Archiving

The sheer explosion of data with the advent of modern scanners. Result in a load of images which necessitates manipulation of data in the Giga byte range along with increasing need for image processing, and graphics at interactive speeds facilitating a high throughput.

Modality	Matrix	No images	File size
Digital mammogram	4092 × 5120 × 12	4	160 MB
Digital radiograph	2048 × 2048 × 12	4	32 MB
CT	512 × 512 × 12	30	15 MB
MRI	256 × 256 × 8	50	6.5 MB
Ultrasound	256 × 256 × 8	24	1.5 MB
Nuclear medicine	128 × 128 × 8	24	0.4 MB

Storage Devices

Medium	Data access for processing
Film	No
Magnetic tape	Yes
Floppy disc	Yes
Magnetic disc	Yes
Optical disc	Yes
Server	Yes

FILM PROCESSING AND FILMING

Film Processing

Processing film is a strict science governed by rigid rules of chemical concentration, temperature, time, and physical movement. Whether processing is done by hand or automatically by machine, excellent radiographs require the highest possible degree of consistency and quality control.

Manual Processing and Darkrooms

Manual processing begins with the darkroom. The darkroom should be located in a central location, adjacent to the reading room and a reasonable distance from the exposure area. For portability darkrooms are often mounted on pickups or trailers.

Film should be located in a light tight compartment, which is most often a metal bin that is used to store and protect the film. An area next to the film bin that is dry and free of dust and dirt should be used to load and unload the film. While another area, the wet side, will be used to process the film. Thus, protecting the film from any water or chemicals that may be located on the surface of the wet-side.

Each of step in film processing must be done properly to develop the image, wash out residual processing chemicals, and to provide adequate shelf-life of the radiograph. The objective of processing is two-fold. First to produce a radiograph adequate for viewing, and secondly to prepare the radiograph for archival storage. A radiograph may be retrieved after 5 or even 20 years in storage.

Automatic Processor Evaluation

The automatic processor is the essential piece of equipment in every X-ray department. The automatic processor will reduce film processing time when compared to manual development by a factor of four. To monitor the performance of a processor, apart from optimum temperature and mechanical checks, chemical and sensitometric checks should be performed for developer and fixer. Chemical checks involve measurement of pH values for developer and replenisher, fixer and replenisher, measurement of specific gravity and fixer silver levels. Ideally pH should be measured daily and it is important to record these measurements, as regular logging provides very useful information. The daily measurements of pH values for developer and fixer can then be plotted to observe the trend of variations in these values compared to normal pH operating levels to identify problems.

Sensitometric checks may be carried out to evaluate if the performance of films in the automatic processors is being maximized. These checks involve measurement of basic fog level, speed and average gradient made at $1°$ C intervals of temperature. The range of temperature measurement depends on the type of chemistry in use, whether cold or hot developer. These three measurements: fog level, speed, and average gradient, should then be plotted against temperature and compared with the manufacturer's supplied figures.

FILM DISPATCH

- Check modality if there is common printing for all modalities.
- Patient data, study data—plain or contrast.
- Exam date/time.
- Number of films.
- Verification of payment.
- Signature from the recipient of the film.

Chapter 2

Development of Scanner Technology

ALL X-RAY CT SYSTEMS USE

- Thinly collimated X-ray beam
- Multiple views
- Detectors to collect X-ray photons
- Data acquisition system
- Image reconstruction algorithm
- Film/monitors to display axial slices

BASIC DIFFERENCE BETWEEN CONVENTIONAL AND HELICAL SCANNERS

Conventional

Tube rotates around stationary patient
(Table is incremented between acquisitions)

- All views in a slice are at same table position
- Power to X-ray tube via cord
- Scan CW and CCW to wind/unwind cord
- Interscan delays:
  3.5 seconds between slices

Helical Scan

Continuous tube rotation—No interscan delays
(Power to X-ray tube via slip ring)

- Continuous table motion as tube rotates
- Each view is at a different table position
  Form images by synthesizing projection data via interpolation

First Generation (Fig. 2.1)

- Single detector
- Translate-rotate acquisition
  — Translates across patient
  — Rotates around patient
- Very slow
  — Minutes per slice

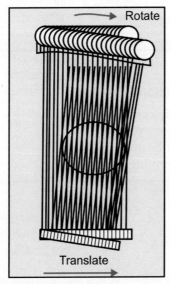

Fig. 2.1: First generation CT scanner

Second Generation (Fig. 2.2)

- Multiple detectors
- Translation-rotation
- Small fan beam
- Shorter scanning times (30 s)

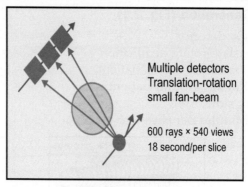

Fig. 2.2: Second generation

Third Generation (Fig. 2.3)

- Multiple detectors
- Rotational movement
- Larger fan beam
- Shorter scanning times (1 to 3 s)

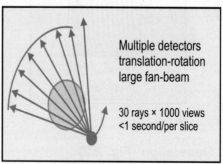

Fig. 2.3: Third generation

Fourth Generation (Fig. 2.4)

- Circular array of fixed detectors (600 to 4800)
- Rotational movement

- Larger fan beam
- Shorter scanning times (1 to 3 s)

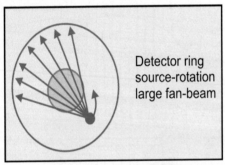

Detector ring
source-rotation
large fan-beam

Fig. 2.4: Fourth generation

Spiral/Helical CT

Simultaneous source rotation, table translation and data acquisition. Projection data for multiple slices covering a volume of the patient, can be aquired at 1 s per slice.

Spiral CT (Fig. 2.5)

The most significant advance in CT technology in the past few years has been the developments of spiral (or helical) CT. During spiral CT, the X-ray tube rotates continuously as the patient is smoothly moved through the X-ray scan field. Unlike the separate data sets produces for each individual slice in standard CT, spiral CT produces one continuous volume set of data for the entire region scanned.

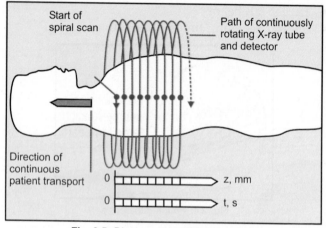

Fig. 2.5: Diagram showing a spiral scan

Spiral CT has Several Advantages Over Standard CT

- *Speed:* Since the patient is moving continuously through the scanner, the duration of the exam is markedly shortened. The entire chest or abdomen can be scanned in 30 seconds, usually during a single breath-hold.
- *Improved detection of small lesions:* In standard CT, the patient holds their breath for a slice acquisition, then breathes, than holds their breath again for the next slice. If they hold their breath slightly differently for each slice, small lesions may fall out of the plane of each contiguous slice and therefore may be missed. Since spiral CT can be performed during a single breath-hold, contiguous slices are truly contiguous. Also, since a volume of data is obtained, the spacing of the acquired slices can be

manipulated after the scan is completed. This allows detected lesions to be placed in the middle of the slice, which creates a more accurate image of the lesion.

- *Improved contrast enhancement:* Intravenous contrast is often injected during the CT scan. Since spiral CT can image a region of interest in such a short period of time, the injection of intravenous contrast can be timed to ensure optimal contrast enhancement and improved evaluation of various organs and blood vessels.

- *Image reconstruction and manipulation:* The volume of data obtained through spiral CT can be manipulated in many fascinating ways by powerful computers connected to the scanner. The transverse images can be reconstructed in any plane. Three dimensional images be formed and moved into any position. A surface view of the body can be created, and then skin, muscles, and overlying organs can be stripped away. Contrast enhanced vessels can be isolated and converted into CT angiograms.

Technical Data for Helical Scans

The fundamental step in helical CT technology is the introduction of slip ring technology. Pioneering work in this field was done by Kalendar in 1989.

Advantages

- Continuous table movement—no interscan delay.
- Image reconstruction at any position or interval.
- Large volume coverage in single breathe hold.
- No interscan delay.

- Form images by synthesising projection data via interpolation.

Spiral Slip Ring

- Also called volumetric, helical, or spiral scanning.
- Allows for the tube and detector components to spin continuously in a non-stop rotation sequence, can scan whole body segments in one breathe hold.

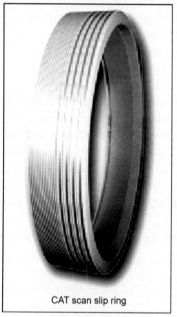

CAT scan slip ring

Fig. 2.6: Slip ring

Reconstruction Principles

Data in spiral CT can be obtained in two ways :

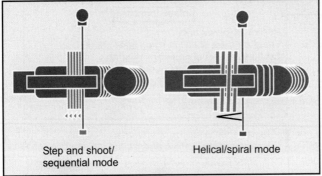

Step and shoot/
sequential mode

Helical/spiral mode

Fig. 2.7: Schematic diagram of tube motion

The major difference in data acquisition in spiral CT is that it displays data from a continuous data stream, that can be computationally manipulated to represent varying amount of projections from adjacent slices thus its possible to reconstruct slices at intervals smaller than the prescribed slice thickness.

This is a major advantage as it helps us to find the best slice through a focal abnormality. It also helps to produce better 3D data sets.

When the acquisition pitch is large and if the reconstruction interval is small not much additional data can be got.

As a thumb rule with a pitch of one—3-5 slices can be reconstructed and with a pitch of 2, two slices can be got.

Effective slice thickness is determined by acquisition parameters (Collimation, pitch) and interpolation

Image formation

Collect projection data
These data are not all at same table position, so:
Synthesize a set of projection data via
interpolation (interpolate between views taken at
same projection angle, but different table positions),
then
Use filtered back projection on synthesized planer data

– Use data 180° each side of reconstruction position
– Introduces artifacts where structure changes along the z-axis

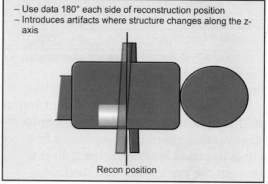

Recon position

Fig. 2.8

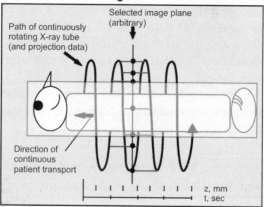

Selected image plane
(arbitrary)

Path of continuously
rotating X-ray tube
(and projection data)

Direction of
continuous
patient transport

z, mm
t, sec

Fig. 2.9: Schematic diagram of helical data interpolation

Pitch

In conventional study the patient is stationary relative to the detector array, while the entire set of projection are needed to reconstruct an image.

In helical scans it is a combination of circular rotation of detectors and simultaneous translation of the patient. Geometrically this combination of rotational and translational movements result in a helecoidal pathway of data projection this raw data has to be first manipulated prior to reconstruction via a process called interpolation among the adjacent projection so that the entire planar data can be reconstructed.

This can be achieved in two ways: 360—interpolation and 180 interpolation, currently the latter is used as it causes least amount of translational distortion and blurring.

Data acquisition
Pitch = $\dfrac{\text{Table movement per rotation}}{\text{Slice collimation}}$
(Essentially a measure of relative speed)
• Contiguous spiral   Pitch = 1 (10 mm / 10 mm)
• Extended (Non-contiguous) spiral   pitch = 2 (20 mm / 20 mm)
• Overlapping spiral   pitch = 1/2 (5 mm / 10 mm)

SUMMARY

Spiral CT - Difference from axial
Image quality (assuming 180 interp. algorithm)

• Effective slice thickness increases with pitch
    (~10% increase for pitch 1; ~30% for pitch 2;
    ~ 70% for pitch 3)
• Hence volume averaging increases with pitch
• Noise is > conventional axial under indentical
    acquisition conditions, but does not change w/ pitch

MULTISLICE SCANNING

As discussed above conventional single slice CT has one X-ray tube and a single row of detectors. The detector row contains 500 to 900 detector elements. In contrast multisection CT has one X-ray tube and multiple rows of detectors. Along the longitudinal axis of the patient. Each row has 500 to 900 detector elements. And many rows together create a two dimensional curved array containing thousands of detector elements. Which are connected to separate data acquisition systems generating multiple channels of separate data.

The use of N detector rows enables us to divide the total X-ray beam into N subdivided beams (the detector row aperture is 1/N of the total X-ray beam collimation). In a multislice CT system, while the total X-ray collimation still indicates the volume coverage speed, the detector row collimation, rather than the total X-ray collimation, determines the z-axis resolution, i.e. the slice thickness. In general, the larger the number of detector rows N, the better the volume coverage speed performance. In the multi-slice CT the ray bundles not only fan out within the gantry plane but also diverge from the gantry plane. This imaging geometry is called the cone-beam imaging geometry, which calls for special cone-beam reconstruction algorithms. Because the scanner discussed has a relatively small number of detector rows and therefore, relatively small cone-beam divergence, parallel fan-beam based reconstruction algorithms can be used to approximate the cone-beam geometry.

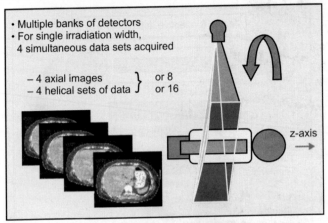

- Multiple banks of detectors
- For single irradiation width, 4 simultaneous data sets acquired

  – 4 axial images   } or 8
  – 4 helical sets of data } or 16

z-axis →

Fig. 2.10: Schematic diagram of multiple detector-geometry

Advantage over single slice

Either same acquisition in shorter time
   or thinner slices for better z-axis resolution
   or scan larger volumes in the same time

Selection of Section Thickness

Selection of thickness by the operator causes:
1. Movement of pre- and post-patient collimation.
2. Selection of detector rows that are combined with the DAS to obtain specified section thickness.

Scanning Speed

Single section CT have a 360° gantry rotation speed of 1 second, multisection scanners can generate 4-16,32 sections per rotation depending upon the speed of the gantry rotation and the number of detectors.

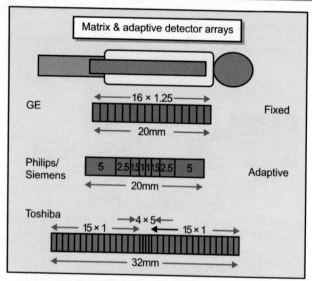

Fig. 2.11: Schematic diagram of detector array configuration

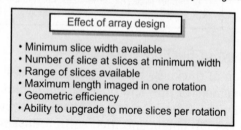

Interpolation algorithms for multislice CT are different from single slice, new type of image distortion which can happen is cone-beam artifact because the beam diverges slightly along the z-axis.

- Improved temporal resolution—faster scanning time results in fewer motion artifacts breathe hold times are reduced.

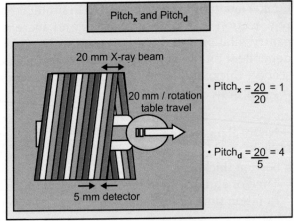

Fig. 2.12: Schematic diagram showing the concept of dual pitch

---

Pitch and multislice image quality

- Z-sensitivity profile width (z-axis resolution)
  – hardly affected by pitch if z-filter interpolation used
- Noise-dose relationship
  – constant with pitch for multi-slice
- Artifacts
  – may be affected by pitch

- Improved spatial resolution—thinner setions improve resolution in the z-axis, reducing partial volume artifacts and increase the diagnostic accuracy.
- Decreased image noise—more patient length is scanned per rotation, thus for extended length study the X-ray tube current can be higher than for single slice. This reduces image noise and improves image resolution.

- Longer anatomic coverage—is due to simultaneous registration of multiple sections and increased gantry rotation speed, the coverage in the z-axis is dependent on the number of data channels, pitch, section thickness, scanning time, and the gantry rotation time.

$$C = n \times p \times s \times t / r$$

N = No. of data channels.
P = Pitch.
S = Section thickness.
T = Time of entire scan in seconds.
R = Rotation time in seconds.

Pitch

Pitch is the parameter without units that provide information about table travel relative to beam collimation. It is defined as table travel per gantry rotation to beam collimation.

In multisection CT two definition of pitch exist because of the confusion caused by some vendors the orginal definition of pitch is preferred because it can be applied to both single and multisection CT without confusion.

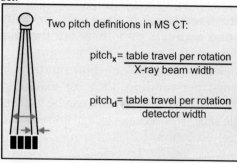

Two pitch definitions in MS CT:

$$\text{pitch}_x = \frac{\text{table travel per rotation}}{\text{X-ray beam width}}$$

$$\text{pitch}_d = \frac{\text{table travel per rotation}}{\text{detector width}}$$

Fig. 2.13

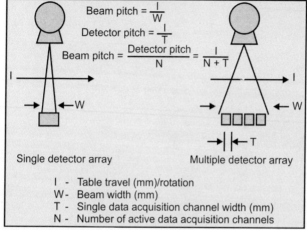

Fig. 2.14: Schematic diagram describing the difference in pitch between single and multislice CT

Isotropic Scanning

Isotropic scanning refers to a situation were mpr images can be created in any plane with the same spatial resolution as the orginal sections for small body parts is resolution is achieved using a small focal spot and scanning with ultra thin sections.

Applications of Multislice CT

Musculoskeletal: with isotropic acquisitions (narrow collimation, lowpitch, high mAs), the quality of multiplanar reformations (MPRS) obtained is very high.
- CT angiography—long coverage possible, without sacrificing spatial resolution,
- Cardiac scoring, brain perfusion, virtual endoscopy, coronary angiography.

Chapter 3

Technical Parameters: In General for All Scanner Types

TECHNICAL PARAMETERS

The quality of the image relates to the fidelity of the CT numbers and to the accurate reproduction of small differences in attenuation (low contrast resolution) and fine detail (spatial resolution). Good imaging performance demands that image quality should be sufficient to meet the clinical requirement for the examination, whilst maintaining the dose to the patient at the lowest level that is reasonably practicable.

In order to achieve this, there must be careful selection of technical parameters that control exposure of the patient and the display of the images, and also regular checking of scanner performance with measurement of physical image parameters as part of a programme of quality assurance.

Display and Exposure Parameters with an Influence on Image Quality and Dose

Nominal Slice Thickness

The slice thickness in CT is a value selected by the operator according to the clinical requirement and generally lies in the range between 1 and 10 mm. In general, the larger the slice thickness, the greater the low contrast resolution in the image; the smaller the slice thickness, the greater the spatial resolution. If the slice thickness is large, the images can be affected by artifact, due to partial volume effects; if the slice thickness is small (e.g. 1-2 mm), the images may be significantly affected by noise.

Inter-slice Distance/Pitch Factor

Inter-slice distance is defined as the couch increment (distance) between two slices. In helical CT the pitch factor is the ratio of the couch increment per rotation to the slice thickness at the axis of rotation. In clinical practice the inter-slice distance generally lies in the range between 2 and 10 mm, and the pitch factor between 1 and 2. In general, for a constant volume of investigation, the smaller the inter-slice distance or pitch factor, the higher both the local dose and the integral dose to the patient. The increase in the local dose is due to superimposition of the dose profiles of the adjacent slices. The increase in the integral dose is due to an increase in the volume of tissue undergoing direct irradiation as indicated by a packing factor.

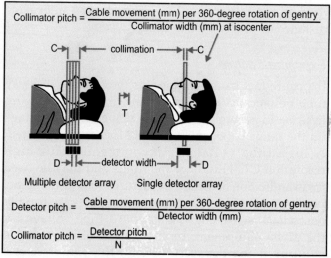

Fig. 3.1: Schematic diagram of pitch

In those cases where 3D reconstruction or reformatting of the images in coronal, sagittal or oblique planes is required, it is necessary to reduce the inter-slice distance to zero or perform a helical scan. In screening or examinations performed with regard to control of disease it can be diagnostically justifiable to have an inter-slice distance corresponding to half the slice thickness or a pitch factor of 1.5 to 2.0.

Volume of Investigation

Volume of investigation, or imaging volume, is the whole volume of the region under examination. It is defined by the outermost margins of the first and last examined slices or helical exposure. The extent of the volume of investigation depends on the clinical needs; in general the greater its value the higher the integral dose to the patient, unless an increased inter-slice distance or pitch factor is used.

Exposure Factors

Exposure factors are defined as the settings of X-ray tube voltage (kV), tube current (mA) and exposure time (s). In general, one to three values of tube voltage (in the range between 80 and 140 kV) can be selected. A high tube voltage is recommended for high resolution CT (HRCT) of the lungs and may be used for examination of osseous structures such as the spine, pelvis and shoulder. Soft tissue structures are usually best visualised using the standard tube voltage for the given equipment. In some cases of quantitative computed tomography (QCT), the same slice is examined with two different values of tube voltage, in order to subtract corresponding images and derive information about the composition of particular tissues. At given values of tube voltage and slice thickness, the image quality depends on the product of X-ray tube current (mA) and exposure time (s), expressed in mAs. Absolute values of mAs necessary for an imaging task will depend on the type of scanner and the patient size and composition. For a particular CT model, an increase in radiographic exposure setting (mAs) is accompanied by a proportional increase in the dose to the patient. Relatively high values of radiographic exposure setting (mAs) should, therefore, be selected only in those cases where a high signal to noise ratio is indispensable.

- Tube potential—80 to 140 kV
  - Voltage between the filaments and anode .
  - Higher potential accelerates electrons more.
  - Tube current—20 to 500 mA.
- Current flowing through the filament.
  - Larger current produces more electrons and greater X-ray beam intensity

Auto mAs option

Some manufacturers have provided this option were the machine automatically selects the optimum mA for a given slice without compromising the image quality resulting in reduced dose.

Principle: This feature requires an ap/lateral scan to obtain information on the X-ray attenuation, so that the mA is increased automatically in areas of high X-ray attenuation.

Field of View

Field of view (FOV) is defined as the maximum diameter of the reconstructed image. Its value can be selected by the operator and generally lies in the range between 12 and 50 cm. The choice of a small FOV allows increased spatial resolution in the image, because the whole reconstruction matrix is used for a smaller region than is the case with a larger FOV; this results in reduction of the pixel size. In any case, the selection of the FOV must take into account not only the opportunity for increasing the spatial resolution but also the need for examining all the areas of possible disease. If the FOV is too small, relevant areas may be excluded from the visible image. If raw data are available the FOV can be changed by post-processing.

Reconstruction parameters

- Reconstruction field of view (10-40 cm)
  - Total size of image in x and y directions
- Reconstruction matrix (usually 512 × 512)
- Convolution kernel /reconstruction filter
  - Variety of filters available from smooth (soft tissue) to sharp (bone)

Gantry Tilt

Gantry tilt is defined as the angle between the vertical plane and the plane containing the X-ray tube, the X-ray beam and the detector array. Its value normally lies in the range between -25° and +25°. The degree of gantry tilt is chosen in each case according to the clinical objective. It may also be used to reduce the radiation dose to sensitive organs or tissues and/or to reduce or eliminate artifacts.

Reconstruction Matrix

Reconstruction matrix is the array of rows and columns of pixels in the reconstructed image, typically 512×512.

Reconstruction Algorithm

Reconstruction algorithm (filter, or kernel) is defined as the mathematical procedure used for the convolution of the attenuation profiles and the consequent reconstruction of the CT image. In most CT scanners, several reconstruction algorithms are available. The appearance and the characteristics of the CT image depend strongly on the algorithm selected. Most CT scanners have special soft tissue or standard algorithms for examination of the head, abdomen, etc. Depending on clinical requirements, it may be necessary to select a high resolution algorithm which provides greater spatial resolution, for detailed representation of bone and other regions of high natural contrast such as pulmonary parenchyma.

Reconstructional Interval

Spiral slice displays data from a continuous data stream, that can be computationally manipulated to represent varying amounts of projections from adjacent slices. Thus, it is possible to reconstruct slices at intervals smaller than the prescribed slice thickness.

If reconstruction interval is small with a large acquisition pitch not much additional data can be obtained.

As a thumb rule 3 to 5 slices can be reconstructed for a pitch of one 2 slices for a pitch of 2.

Finer reconstruction intervals may not prove additional information, even though they may enhance the visual effect of 3D images.

Window Width

Window width is defined as the range of CT numbers converted into grey levels and displayed on the image monitor. It is expressed in HU. The window width can be selected by the operator according to the clinical requirements, in order to produce an image from which the clinical information may be easily extracted. In general, a large window (for instance 400 HU) represents a good choice for acceptable representation of a wide range of tissues. Narrower window widths adjusted to diagnostic requirements are necessary to display details of specific tissues with acceptable accuracy.

Window Level

Window level is expressed in HU and is defined as the central value of the window used for the display of the reconstructed CT image. It should be selected by the viewer according to the attenuation characteristics of the structure under examination.

Clinical and Associated Performance Parameters

A series of clinical factors play a special part in the optimal use of ionising radiation in CT. They are described here in order to ensure that an appropriate CT examination is carried out, providing diagnostic quality with a reasonable radiation dose for the patient.

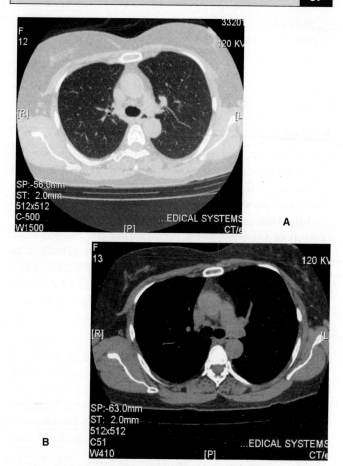

Figs 3.2A and B: Same image set in lung and mediastinal window

A CT examination should, therefore, only be carried out on the basis of a justifiable clinical indication, and exposure of the patient should always be limited to the minimum necessary to meet clinical objectives.

Adequate clinical information, including the records of previous imaging investigations, must be available to the person approving requests for CT.

In certain applications, in order to practice CT effectively, prior investigation of the patient by other forms of imaging might be required.

Supervision

CT examinations should be performed under the clinical responsibility of a radiologist/practitioner according to the regulations and standard examination protocols should be available.

Effective supervision may support radiation protection of the patient by terminating the examination when the clinical requirement has been satisfied, or when problems occurring during the examination (for example, unexpected uncooperation by the patient or the discovery of contrast media residue from previous examinations) cannot be overcome.

Problems and pitfalls: The responsible radiologist/practitioner should be aware of clinical or technical problems which may interfere with image quality. Many of these are particular to specific organs or tissues and may lead to modification of technique. The radiologist/practitioner and the radiographer must be aware of manoeuvres which may be used to overcome such diagnostic or technical problems in order to provide a clinically relevant examination.

Patient Preparation

The following patient-related operational parameters play an important role for the quality of the CT examination:

Cooperation: Patient cooperation should be ensured as far as possible prior to the examination. An explanation of the procedure should be given to each patient. Good communication with and control of the patient is equally necessary during the whole examination.

Protective shielding: Relevant protection for sensitive organs outside the imaging field is a lead-purse for the male gonads, if the edge of the volume of investigation is less than 10-15 cm away. The protection of female gonads by wrap-around lead has not yet been demonstrated. Appropriate protection measures must be applied to persons who, for clinical reasons or to ensure cooperation, may need to accompany patients in the examination room during the examination.

Clothing: The area of examination should be free of external metal or other radio-dense items where possible. Special attention must be given to eliminating any X-ray dense material in the patient's clothes or hair.

Fasting: Fasting prior to the examination is not essential. Restraint from food, but not fluid, is recommended if intravenous contrast media are to be given.

Intravenous contrast media: These are needed in some examinations and must be employed in a manner appropriate to the clinical indication, taking into consideration the risk factors.

Oral or cavitatory contrast media: Oral contrast medium may be required in abdomino-pelvic examinations and must be administered at times and in doses appropriate to the indication. Administration of contrast medium per rectum may be required in some examinations of the pelvis and a vaginal tampon should be used in some examinations for gynaecological applications.

Positioning and motion: Most CT examinations are carried out with the patient supine. In this position the patient is most comfortable with the knees flexed. Alternate positioning may be required to aid comfort and cooperation, for appropriate display of anatomy, to reduce absorbed radiation to particular organs, or to minimise artifact. Motion should be kept to a minimum to reduce artifacts; typical sources of artifacts are involuntary patient movement, respiration, cardiovascular action, peristalsis and swallowing.

Examination Technique

Scanogram
A scanogram permits the examination to be planned and controlled accurately, and provides a record of the location of images. It is recommended that this is performed in all cases. In general such imaging provides only a small fraction of the total patient dose during a complete CT procedure.

Clinical aspects of setting the appropriate technical parameters.
These parameters must be set according to the area of examination and clinical indication, as follows:
- Nominal slice thickness is chosen according to the size of the anatomical structure or lesion that needs to be visualised. Staff should be aware of the implications of choice of slice thickness in relation to the image quality and radiation dose to the patient.

- Inter-slice distance is chosen according to the area under examination and the clinical indication. Staff should be aware of the risk of overlooking lesions which fall in the inter-slice interval during serial CT. In general, the interval should not exceed one half of the diameter of suspected lesions. This problem is absent in helical scanning, when an appropriate reconstruction index is used.
- Field of view (FOV). Selection of FOV must respect image resolution and the need to examine all areas of possible disease. If the FOV is too small, disease may be excluded from the visible image.
- *Exposure factors:* Tube voltage (kV), tube current (mA) and exposure time (s) affect image quality and patient dose. Increasing exposure increases low contrast resolution by reducing noise but also increases patient dose. Patient size is an important factor in determining the image noise. Image quality consistent with the clinical indications should be achieved with the lowest possible dose to the patient. In certain examinations image noise is a critical issue and higher doses might be required.
- The volume of investigation is the imaging volume, defined by the beginning and end of the region imaged. It should cover all regions of possible disease for the particular indication.
- *Reconstruction algorithm:* This is set according to the indication and area under examination. For most examinations, images are displayed utilising algorithms suitable for soft tissues; other algorithms available include those providing greater spatial resolution for detailed display of bone and other areas of high natural contrast.

Helical or Spiral CT

- The repeating of single scans, which sometimes results from lack of patient cooperation in serial CT, is reduced in spiral CT because of the shorter examination times involved.
- For pitch >1 the dose will be reduced compared with contiguous serial scanning; there are no data missing as may be the case with the use of an inter-slice interval in serial CT.
- The practice of using overlapping scans or thin slices in serial CT for high quality 3D display or multi-planar reconstructions is replaced by the possibility of reconstructing overlapping images from one helical scan volume data set.
- Extremely shortened examination time:
  - Makes it possible to acquire continuous patient data during a single breath-hold; problems with inconsistent respiration can thereby be avoided.
  - Disturbances due to involuntary movements such as peristalsis and cardiovascular action are reduced.
  - May optimize scanning with the use of intra-venous contrast media.
- Images can be reconstructed for any couch position in the volume of investigation:
  - Anatomical misregistration is avoided.
  - Equivocal lesions can be further evaluated without additional patient exposure.
  - The possibility of displaying the data volume in transverse slices reconstructed at intervals smaller than the X-ray beam collimation results in overlapping slices which, in combination with

reduced or eliminated movement artifacts, makes it possible to perform high quality three-dimensional (3D) and multi-planar reconstructions with smooth tissue contours. This is used especially in skeletal and vascular imaging (CT angiography).

Helical CT, however, has drawbacks such as:

- Ease of performance may tempt the operator to extend the examination unjustifiably, either by increasing the imaging volume, or by repeated exposure of a region.
- Although most image quality parameters are equivalent for contiguous serial CT and helical CT performed with a pitch = 1, the performance of helical CT with a pitch greater than 1.5 may imply lower and possibly insufficient diagnostic image quality due to reduced low contrast resolution
- Spatial resolution in the z-direction is lower than indicated by the nominal slice width unless special interpolation is performed.
- The technique has inherent artifact.

When using helical CT in conjunction with intravenous injection of contrast media to provide optimally enhanced images, careful timing of exposure relative to intravenous injection is mandatory.

Image Viewing Conditions

It is recommended that initial reading of CT images is carried out from the TV monitor. Display of images and post-processing image reconstruction should be at a display matrix of at least 512×512.

Brightness and contrast control on the viewing monitor should be set to give a uniform progression of the grey-scale from black to white. A calibrated grey-scale would be preferable.

Settings of window width and window level dictate the visible contrast between tissues and should generally be chosen to give optimum contrast between normal structures and lesions.

Film Processing

Optimal processing of the film has important implications for the diagnostic quality of the image stored on film. Film processors should be maintained at their optimum operating conditions as determined by the manufacturer and by regular and frequent quality control procedures.

Physical Parameters: Physical Measures of Scanner Performance

The quality of the CT image may be expressed in terms of physical parameters such as uniformity, linearity, spatial resolution, low contrast resolution and absence of artifacts according to IEC recommendations. It depends on the technological characteristics of the CT scanner, the exposure factors used and image viewing conditions. Quality may be assessed by quantitative measurement of the parameters listed above, using suitable test phantoms, and by the appearance of artifacts. These measurements should be conducted regularly, in order to guarantee the maintenance of performance of the CT scanner during its whole period of use. It is essential that such technical quality control has been performed when using the criteria presented in these guidelines.

Test Phantoms

Test phantoms (phantom of a standardised human shape or test objects of a particular shape, size and structure) are used for the purposes of calibration and evaluation of the performance of CT scanners. Performance is checked by acceptance tests after installation and important repairs, and by periodic quality control tests, as established in standardised protocols. A number of test phantoms are commercially available and most manufacturers provide one or more test objects.

The test phantoms should allow for the following parameters to be checked: mean CT number, uniformity, noise, spatial resolution, slice thickness, dose and positioning of couch.

CT Number

The accuracy of CT number is verified by scanning a test object utilising the usual operating parameters and reconstruction algorithms. The CT number is affected by the X-ray tube voltage, beam filtration and object thickness. The CT number of water is by definition equal to 0 HU and the mean CT number measured over the central region of interest (ROI) should be in the range +/- 4 HU.

Linearity

Linearity concerns the linear relationship between the calculated CT number and the linear attenuation coefficient of each element of the object. It is essential for the correct evaluation of a CT image and, in particular, for the accuracy of QCT. Deviations from linearity should not exceed +/- 5 HU over specific ranges (soft tissue or bone).

Uniformity

Uniformity relates to the requirement for the CT number of each pixel in the image of a homogeneous object to be the same within narrow limits over various regions of the object such as a cylindrical 20 cm diameter phantom of water-equivalent plastic. The difference in the mean CT number between a peripheral and a central region of a homogeneous test object should be $\leq$ 8 HU. Such differences are largely due to the physical phenomenon of beam hardening.

Noise

Picture element (pixel) or image noise is the local statistical fluctuation in the CT numbers of individual picture elements of a homogeneous ROI. Noise is dependent on the radiation dose and has a marked effect on low contrast resolution. The magnitude of the noise is indicated by the standard deviation of the CT numbers over a ROI in a homogeneous substance. It should be measured over an area of about 10% of the cross-sectional area of the test object. Image noise diminishes with the use of a slightly flattened convolution kernel, with simultaneous reduction of spatial resolution and an increase in low contrast resolution. Image noise is inversely proportional to the square root of the dose and to the slice thickness. For example, if the dose is halved then the noise will only increase by about 40 percent. Conversely, a reduction in slice thickness requires a proportionate increase in dose in order to avoid an increase in noise. The medical problem under study and the corresponding image quality required should determine what level of image noise and what patient dose are reasonably practicable.

Spatial Resolution

Spatial resolution at high and low contrast are interdependent and critical to image quality and good imaging of diagnostically important structures.

The spatial resolution at high contrast (high contrast resolution) determines the minimum size of detail visualised in the plane of the slice with a contrast >10 percent. It is affected by the reconstruction algorithm, the detector width, the slice thickness, the object to detector distance, the X-ray tube focal spot size, and the matrix size.

The spatial resolution at low contrast (low contrast resolution) determines the size of detail that can be visibly reproduced when there is only a small difference in density relative to the surrounding area. Low contrast resolution is considerably limited by noise. The perception threshold in relation to contrast and detail size can be determined, for example, by means of a contrast-detail curve. In such determinations, the effects of the reconstruction algorithm and of the other scanning parameters have to be known. Dose and the corresponding image noise greatly affect low contrast resolution.

Slice Thickness

The slice thickness is determined in the centre of the field of view as the distance between the two points on the sensitivity profile along the axis of rotation at which response has fallen to 50 percent. Certain deviations in thickness should not be exceeded because of the effect of slice thickness on image detail; for example, with a nominal slice thickness > 8 mm, a maximum deviation of ± 10 percent is acceptable; tolerable deviations for smaller slice thickness of 2 to 8 mm and < 2 mm are ± 25 percent and ± 50 percent, respectively.

The use of post-patient collimation, which is inherent in some CT equipment to reduce the slice sensitivity profile, leads to significant increases in the patient dose for a series of contiguous slices.

Stability of CT Numbers

Stability is defined as the maintenance overtime of constancy of CT number and of uniformity. It can be checked by means of a suitable test object, containing at least three specimens of different materials, e.g. water, Polymethyl-methacrylate (PMMA) and Teflon. Deviations should not exceed +/- 5 CT numbers with respect to initial mean values. A similar tolerance should be applied in the verification of uniformity, as measured in three ROIs, each containing approximately

100 pixels and placed respectively at the centre, at the periphery, and in a position intermediate between the centre and the periphery of the reconstructed image.

Positioning of Couch

The accuracy of positioning of the patient couch is evaluated by moving the loaded couch a defined distance relative to the gantry and subsequently moving it back to the start position. Positional accuracy includes both deviation in longitudinal positioning and also backlash. Maximum tolerances of ±2 mm apply to both criteria. These also apply to mobile CT equipment.

Image Quality Modification Based on the Clinical Requirement

High Signal to Noise

- Useful in lung nodule characterization.
- COPD.
- Coronary artery calcification.

Low Signal to Noise Task

- Abdominal scans.
- Diffuse lung disease.

Medium Signal to Noise Task

- Brain.
- Paediatric scans.

Chapter 4

Practical Overview of Performing a CT Scan

PATIENT POSITIONING 1

The scan procedure start with patient positioning within the gantry, the parts of the gantry is showed, although the design of machines vary between the manufacturers the basic principles remain the same.
- Image quality starts with proper positioning.
- Poor patient positioning cause artifacts.

MAIN COMPONENTS

Gantry

Function

The gantry incorporates the X-ray tube unit, the high-light detector and DAS (Data acquisition system) inside. It also provides the following functions.
- *Display panel:* The display shows the reading of the gentry tilt, table height, position of landmark, latch status, scannable range and tilt range.

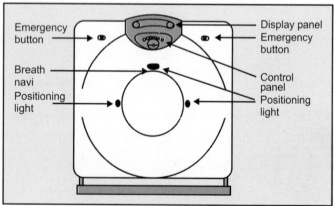

Fig. 4.1: Diagram of CT scan gantry

- *Emergency button:* Pressing the emergency button stops every mechanical movement and the X-ray emission.
- *Control panel:* The control panel incorporates the several buttons to mainly control the movements of the gantry and table. Each front and rear cover has two control panels.
- *Positioning light and breath navi:* The Halogen will be emitted through here that will be used to position a patient breath navi gives the visual breathing instructions to a patient with hearing problem.

Table

Function

The table is used to load a patient for scanning.

- *Cradle:* The cradle moves into or out of the gantry aperture.
- *Latch button:* The latch button is used to latch or unlatch the cradle. The unlatched cradle can be manually slid. The display panel shows whether the cradle is latched.
- *Speaker:* The speaker is used to deliver oral instructions to a patient.
- *Mat switch:* The mat switch is placed at the foot of the table. When the operator steps on it, the switch turns on and activates functional buttons on the gantry panel.

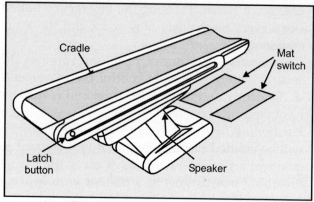

Fig. 4.2: Diagram of a CT scan couch

Operator Console (OC)

Function

The operator console (OC) is mainly used for the operator to set up the scan procedures and process the resultant image data.

- *Scan/display monitor:* The 17 inch monitor (21 inch optional) on the OC can be mainly used for two purposes, scanning patients and displaying images.
- *Keyboard/Mouse:* Please refer to the User Interface on page 1-10
- *Main switch:* Please refer to the System power On/Off on page 1-22
- *CD-ROM drive:* This drive is dedicated to service of application software installation.
- *MOD (Magnetic Optical Disk) drive (optional):* Image data can be stored in 5 inch MOD.

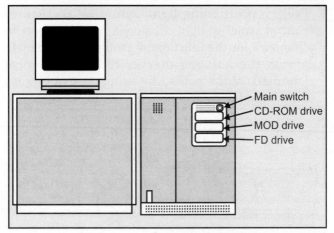

Fig. 4.3: Diagram of CT scan console

Caution: It is highly recommended to always take back-up image data because of a possibility of medium breakdown.

PATIENT POSITIONING 2

1. In order to safely lay a patient on the cradle, make sure first that the cradle is locked.

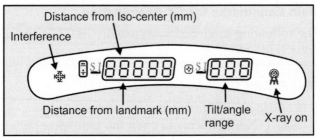

Fig. 4.4: Diagram of gantry display panel

2. Press a positioning light button on the gantry control panel to light a halogen marker (Refer to chapter 1 for the function of gantry control panel).
3. Match the halogen marker to an anatomical landmark of the patient by using control buttons on the gantry control panel.

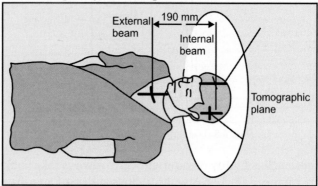

Fig. 4.5: Diagram depicting tomographic planes

Patient positioning ends when the table location figure is displayed on the display panel.

PATIENT POSITIONING 3

Main Landmarks for CT Examination

The following landmarks are usually in CT examinations (Fig. 4.6).

New Patient 1

Select (new patient) to initiate a new examination.
1. Select (New patient) to open the following patient information/protocol selection screen.

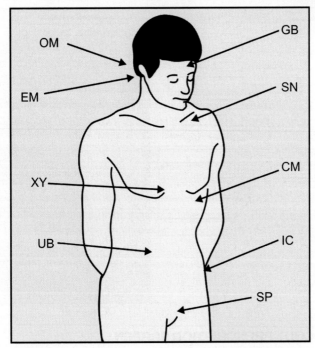

Fig. 4.6: Diagram showing normal landmarks for positioning

GB: Glabella
EM: External auditory meatus
XY: Xyphoid
IC: Iliac crest
SP: Symphysis pubis

OM: Orbital meatal line
SN: Sternal notch
CM: Costal margin
UB: Umbilicus

2. Enter the patient demographic data.
   Note: As a minimum, the patient ID must be entered
   – Exam number: (within 12 characters)
   – Accession number: (within 16 characters)
   – Patient ID: (within 16 characters)
   – Patient's name: (within 64 characters)

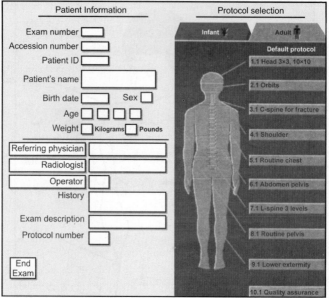

Fig. 4.7: Sample scout of CT/ₑ GE scanner

SCOUT PRESCRIPTION SCREEN

Axial/Helical Scan Prescription 1

Axial/Helical Prescription (View/Edit) Screen

After scout scan, you may proceed to the following axial/helical prescription screen to perform axial, helical or cine scans.

- *Image area:* Images will be displayed here. This image area can be enlarged to full screen by clicking on the small square icon located in the upper right corner.
- *Prior/Next:* Prior or next key appears on the screen only when more than three groups are prescribed.

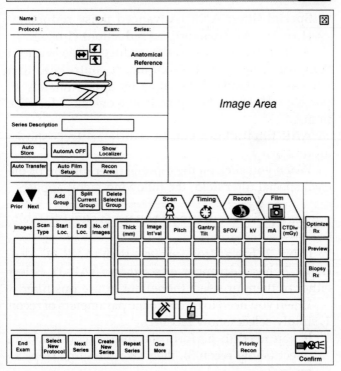

Fig. 4.8: Sample page for planning act study from CT/e GE scanner

SCAN RECONSTRUCTION PARAMETERS

Prospective Multiple Reconstruction

- Recon type: Soft, STND, STD+, DETL, chest, bone edge or PERM
- Image filters: Smooth (S1, S11, S2, S21, S3), Edge (E1, E2, E21, E22, E23), Lung (L1, L2, L3)
- Matrix size: 256 × 256, 320 × 320 or 512 × 512
- Motion correct: Motion correction

- Special filter: ANR (Advanced noise reduction) (1 or 2) AAR (Arm artifact reduction) (1 or 2)

ANR filter allows you to reduce noise without compromising spatial resolution. It contributes to a decrease in standard deviation by approximately 10 percent which may be equivalent to one-step decrease in mA.

AAR filter allows you to reduce artifacts shown around arms.

When you click on the (Special filter) button or the each special filter field, the following menu appears.

None	ANR 1	ANR 2	AAR 1	AAR 2	Cancel

(ANR 2) has a stronger effect than (ANR 1). Also, (AAR 2) has a stronger effect than (AAR 1). Select either of them or select (none) not to use this filter.

When you need to return to the parameters of recon 1, simply select (show recon 1),

1. If you need to perform the third reconstruction, select (show recon 3), then take the same steps as recon 2.
2. Select (Confirm) to intiate a scan.

Note: During the scan, only the set of recon 1 will be reconstructed. In order to activate recon 2 or 3, select any of the following buttons (end exam), (create new series), (next series), (select new protocol) or (repeat series).

Technique

Generation of scout images: Patient lies supine on scanning couch and is advanced towards the scanning field in the gantry. A scout film is generated by generating the X-ray beam and passing the relevant part of the patient in one movement through the gantry.

This continuous exposure as the patient moves through the beam generates a topogram resembling an X-ray from the scout the position number and angulation of the subsequent slices are chosen.

Imaging Planes

- *Axial*—advantage of direct right-left comparison. Ease of performance.
- *Coronal*—geometric advantage of offering scans at right angles to major bone structures. Helps to clarify the relationship of a lesion seen in axial sections.
- *Sagittal*—useful for assessing midline structures. Usually a reformatted projection as direct sagittal aquisition is anatomically difficult to obtain.

Chapter 5

Image Acquisition Protocols

Protocols are guidelines used to scan a particular area of interests, they are flexible and should be adapted to suit the patient. Parameters used are not rigid and can be changed when appropriate. Used as a tool to reduce radiation dose.

FACTORS TO BE CONSIDERED FOR SCAN PLANNING

- Positioning and scout.
- Type of scan—axial or helical.
- Slice thickness.
- Increment of gantry movement.
- Exposure factors—kVp, mAs.
- Field of view.
- Pitch.
- Contrast consideration.

Slice Thickness

- Slice thickness is determined by beam collimation, size thickness is dependent on the size of the detectors and is usually about 10 mm.
- Thin slices produce better spatial resolution.
- Radiation dose in CT is inversely proportional to slice thickness.

Incrementation

- Incrementation is defined as the distance between scans.
- The starting point of the scan is defined as 0, distance is measured from this location as S or I (superior or inferior).

- In helical scans the image increments may be changed after the scan has been completed.
- Overlapping scans can be used for 3D reformations, small lesions are to be displayed.

Field of View

- Determines the size of the image on the screen.
- From a given FOV, FOV may be changed smaller after completion of scan, but cannot be changed to larger.
- Technologist should select FOV to suit the patient and anatomy.
- Small FOV enhances the spatial resolution.

Exposures

- kVp defines the quality of the beam.
- Higher kVp is needed for penetration of thick anatomy.
- Thin sections require higher kVp so as to improve the signal to noise ratio.
- mAs defines the quantity of the beam.
- Low mAs will degrade the image.
- High mAs will increase the heat generation and decrease the life of the scan.
- Patient dose is increased with increased mAs.

Pitch

- It is defined as the ratio of the speed of table to the slice thickness.
- Higher pitch reduces the scan time.

- If the table moves exactly the same as slice thickness through one tube rotation, the pitch is said to be one.
- Pitch of 2 means the table moves a total of 2x the slice thickness which results in a faster scan.

CRANIUM
- Brain, general
- Skull base
- CT angiography.

FACE AND NECK
- Face and sinuses
- Petrous bone
- Orbits
- Sella and hypophysis
- Salivary glands (Parotid and submandibular)
- Pharynx
- Larynx.

SPINE
- Vertebral and paravertebral structures
- Lumbar spine, discal herniation.

CHEST
- Chest, general
- Chest, mediastinal vessels
- Chest, HRCT (High Resolution Computed Tomography).

ABDOMEN AND PELVIS

- Abdomen, general
- Liver and spleen
- Kidneys
- Pancreas
- Adrenal glands
- Pelvis, general.

BONES AND JOINTS

- Osseous pelvis
- Shoulder joint
- Elbow joints
- Wrist
- Hip
- Knee
- Ankle.

CT Brain

Indication: Trauma, cerebrovascular accidents, seizures, congenital lesions, meningitis.

Patient preparation: Information about the procedure; restraint from food, but not fluid, is recommended, if intravenous contrast media are to be given.

Scanogram: Lateral scano from vertex to maxilla.

Image criteria: Visualization of all brain structures, skull base and sinus if needed.

FOV: Head dimension (about 24 cm).

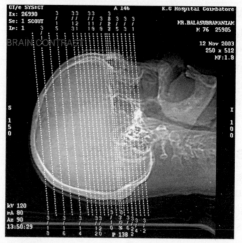

Fig. 5.1: Digital scanogram showing slice planning for brain

Gantry tilt: 0 to −10° from OM for axial scanning.
- *X-ray tube voltage (kV):* Standard
- *Tube current and exposure time product (mAs):* Should be as low as consistent with required image quality
- *Reconstruction algorithm:* Standard
- *Window width:* 1500-3000 HU (bones)140-1000 HU (soft tissue)
- *Window level:* 200-400 HU (bones)30-100 HU (soft tissue).

IV contrast: 40 ml of ionic/nonionic contrast.

Circle of Willis: R/O Aneurysm

Specific anatomic region: Circle of Willis.

Application: R/O aneurysm.

Injection rate: 3 ml/sec

Contrast volume and type: 90 ml of nonionic contrast.

Area scanned: Entire brain (with a single box over the circle of Willis area s5- s40 table position).

Scan delay: Usually 15-20 sec.

Length of spiral (time): 40 sec.

Slice thickness: 1 mm.

Table speed/pitch: 1.

Reconstruction Interval: 0.5 mm.

3D technique used: Mip/volume rendering .

FACE AND SINUSES

Indications: Trauma, malformations, malignancies and inflammation.

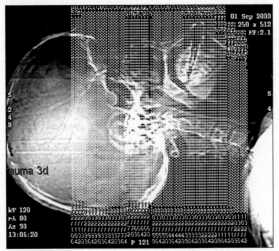

Fig. 5.2: Digital scanogram showing slice planning for face

...ary investigations: Appropriate X-ray exami-
...on of the face except for isolated evaluation of the sinuses.

Patient preparation: Information about the procedure; restraint from food, but not fluid, is recommended, if intravenous contrast media are to be given.

Scan projection radiograph: Lateral from jaw to vertex.

Image Criteria
- Visualization of entire face from palate to the top of the frontal sinus.
- Vessels after intravenous contrast media.

FOV: Head dimension (about 24 cm).

Gantry tilt: 0 to −10° from OM for axial scanning of the face; according to the patient position for coronal scanning.

X-ray tube voltage (kV): Standard.

Tube current and exposure time product (mAs): Should be as low as consistent with required image quality.

Reconstruction algorithm: High resolution or standard.

Window width: 1500-3000 HU (bones), 140-1000 HU (soft tissue).

Window level: 200-400 HU (bones), 30-100 HU (soft tissue).

Pitfalls: Artifacts from teeth or dental prothesis/ fillings.

Modification to technique: Change of gantry angulation or patient position to avoid artifact.

Examination of the sinuses in a prone position to keep inflammatory secretion away from the osteomeatal complex.

Examination of the sinuses for functional endoscopic sinus surgery is best performed directly in the coronal plane.

IV contrast— 60–120 ml of ionic/nonionic contrast based on the indication.

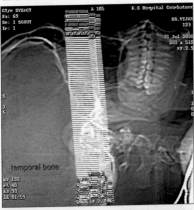

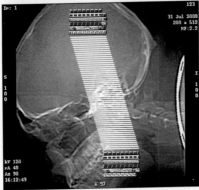

Figs 5.3A and B: Axial and coronal digital scanograms showing slice pan for temporal lobe

PETROUS TEMPORAL BONE

Indications: Hearing deficits, inflammation, vertigo, facial or acoustic nerve diseases, malformations, bone diseases and trauma.

Preliminary investigations: Examination of acoustic and labyrinth function, evoked potentials; appropriate X-ray examination of skull, base and petrous bone may only occasionally be necessary.

Patient preparation: Information about the procedure; restraint from food, but not fluid, is recommended, if intravenous contrast media are to be given.

Scan projection radiograph: Lateral from mastoid to above skull base.

Image Criteria

- Visualization of entire petrous bone.
- Vessels after intravenous contrast media.

Patient position: Supine, for axial scans; supine or prone for coronal scans.

Volume of investigation: From 0.5 cm below to 0.5 cm above the petrous bone.

Nominal slice thickness: 1-3 mm.

Inter-slice distance/pitch: Contiguous or a pitch = 1.0.

FOV: Head dimension (about 24 cm); secondary reduction of FOV is necessary for evaluation of subtle pathology.

Gantry tilt: OM line or tilted above OM line for axial scanning; according to the patient position for coronal scanning.

X-ray tube voltage (kV): Standard.

Tube current and exposure time product (mAs): Should be as low as consistent with required image quality.

Reconstruction algorithm: High resolution or standard.

Window width: 2000-3000 HU (bones)140-160 HU (soft tissue)1500-2500 HU (middle setting).

Window level: 200-400 HU (bones)30-40 HU (soft tissue)150-250 HU (middle setting).

Pitfalls:
- Calcifications versus contrast enhancement Interpetrous bone hardening artifacts.

Modification to technique:
- Subtle irregularity can be checked with slices in the area of suspected pathology, before considering contrast administration
- Higher mAs may be required if artifacts degrade the image quality in the posterior fossa
- Coronal scans may be used to reduce artifacts.

IV contrast—40-80 ml ionic/nonionic agents based on indication.

ORBITS

Indications: Structural diseases of the orbits and orbital content, trauma, foreign body.

*Advisable preliminary investigations:*Evaluation of visual function; evoked potentials; appropriate X-ray examination of the orbits may occasionally be necessary.

Patient preparation: Information about the procedure; restraint from food, but not fluid, is recommended, if intravenous contrast media are to be given.

Scan projection radiograph: Lateral from jaw to vertex.

Image criteria:
Visualization of
• Entire orbits
• Osseous walls
• Vessels after intravenous contrast media

Patient position: Supine for axial scans; supine or prone for coronal scans.

Volume of investigation: From 0.5 cm below to 0.5 cm above the orbital cavity.

Nominal slice thickness: 2-5 mm.

Inter-slice distance/pitch: Contiguous or a pitch = 1.0.

FOV: Head dimension (about 24 cm); secondary reduction of FOV is necessary for evaluation of subtle pathology.

Gantry tilt: -6 to -10° from OM or parallel to the optic nerve for axial scanning; according to the patient position for coronal scanning.

X-ray tube voltage (kV): Standard.

Tube current and exposure time product (mAs): Should be as low as consistent with required image quality.

Reconstruction algorithm: High resolution or standard

Window width: 140-300 HU (soft tissue), 2000-3000 HU (bones), about 4000 HU (special orbit window).

Window level: 30-40 HU (soft tissue), 200-400 HU (bones), about 0 HU (special orbit window).

Motion: Movement artifact deteriorates image quality (prevented by head fixation or sedation of non-cooperative patients).

Intravenous contrast media: Useful to identify vascular structures and enhancing lesions.

Pitfalls
- Calcifications versus contrast enhancement
- Foreign bodies (beam hardening artifacts)
- Artifacts from orbital or dental prothesis/fillings.

Modification to technique: Change of gantry angulation or patient position to avoid artifact.

IV contrast: 40-60 ml based on indication.

SELLA

Indications: Suspicion of sellar or hypophyseal alterations (endocrinological diseases, visual defects, alterations of ocular motility).

Scan projection radiograph: Lateral from C2 to above skull base.

Image criteria:
Visualization of:
- Entire hypophyseal region including osseous walls
- Vessels after intravenous contrast media.

Patient position: Supine for axial scans; supine or prone for coronal scans.

Volume of investigation: From 0.5 cm below to 0.5 cm above the hypophyseal region.

Nominal slice thickness: 2-3 mm.

Inter-slice distance/pitch: Contiguous or a pitch = 1.0.

FOV: Head dimension (about 24 cm); secondary reduction of FOV is necessary for evaluation of subtle pathology.

Gantry tilt: OM line for axial scanning; according to the patient position for coronal scanning.

X-ray tube voltage (kV): Standard.

Tube current and exposure time product (mAs): Should be as low as consistent with required image quality.

Reconstruction algorithm: Soft tissue or high resolution.

Window width: 140-300 HU (soft tissue), 2000-3000 HU (bones).

Window level: 30-40 HU (soft tissue), 200-400 HU (bones)

Pitfalls:
- Foreign bodies (beam hardening artifacts)
- Artifacts from dental prothesis/fillings.

Modification to technique: Change of gantry angulation or patient position to avoid artifact.

IV contrast: 50-80 ml based on indication.

PHARYNX

Indications: Diagnosis of parapharyngeal masses; T/N staging of pharyngeal neoplasms.

Advisable preliminary investigations: Endoscopy may be performed.

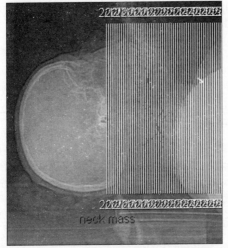

neck mass

Fig. 5.4: Digital scanogram showing slice plane for pharynx

Patient preparation: Information about the procedure; restraint from food, but not fluid, is recommended, if intravenous contrast media are to be given.

Scan projection radiograph: Lateral from orbital roof to root of neck.

Image criteria:
Visualization of:
- Entire pharynx
- Regional lymph node areas and associated muscles
- Base of the skull
- Esophagopharyngeal junction
- Vessels after intravenous contrast media.

Patient position: Supine.

Volume of investigation: Nasopharynx: from sphenoid bone to hyoid bone and continue to root of the neck for N-staging of neoplasms; oropharynx/hypopharynx: from palate to root of the neck.

Nominal slice thickness: 3-5 mm serial or preferably helical.

Inter-slice distance/pitch: Contiguous, but for large lesions distances of < 3-5 mm or a pitch up to 1.5-2.0 may be used.

FOV: Adjusted to the minimum required to demonstrate complete cross-section of the face. Reduction of FOV may be necessary for the evaluation of subtle pathologies.

Gantry tilt: None.

X-ray tube voltage (kV): Standard.

Tube current and exposure time product (mAs): Should be as low as consistent with image quality.

Reconstruction algorithm: Soft tissue/standard or if necessary high resolution.

Window width: 300-500 HU.

Window level: 0-30 HU (unenhanced examination), 30-60 HU (enhanced examination).

Pitfalls:
- Artifact from dental prothesis/fillings
- Apposition of the pharyngeal mucosal folds may obscure pathology
- Pooling of saliva may mimic pathology
- Superficial mucosal extent of neoplasms may not be identified
- Secretion from oropharyngeal neoplasms.

Modification to technique: Intrathecal injection of contrast medium (CT myelography) to delineate the spinal cord and nerve roots (nonionic contrast 8-10 ml).

CHEST, MEDIASTINAL VESSELS

Indications: Suspected or known major vessel aneurysm, dissection or congenital anomaly.

Advisable preliminary investigations: Chest radiography, including lateral projection.

Patient preparation: Information about the procedure; restraint from food, but not fluid, is recommended, if intravenous contrast media are to be given.

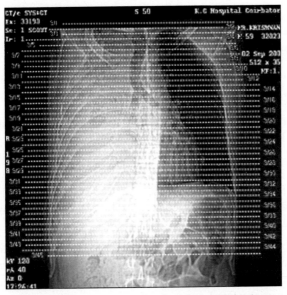

Fig. 5.5: Digital scanogram showing slice plane for thorax

Scan projection radiograph: Frontal from neck to upper abdomen.

Image criteria:
Visualization of:
- Entire thoracic aorta
- Entire vena cava
- Entire heart
- Vessels after intravenous contrast media
- Patient position: supine, arms above the head.

Volume of investigation: May be limited to area of radiographic abnormality or clinically suspected lesion.

Nominal slice thickness: 4-5 mm serial or preferably helical.

Inter-slice distance/pitch: Contiguous or a pitch = 1.0; 2-4 mm or a pitch up to 1.2 - 1.5 for large lesions.

FOV: Limited to area of the heart and major vessels.

Gantry tilt: None.

X-ray tube voltage (kV): Standard.

Tube current and exposure time product (mAs): Should be as low as consistent with required image quality.

Reconstruction algorithm: Soft tissue/standard.

Window width: 100-400 HU (soft tissue, unenhanced examination) 150-500 HU (soft tissue, enhanced examination).

Window level: 0-50 HU (soft tissue, unenhanced examination) 20-150 HU (soft tissue, enhanced examination, depends on dose and method of contrast administration).

Problems and pitfalls:
- Artifact from the cardiac outline may cross the aorta and mimic dissection flap
- Inhomogeneities in luminal opacification due to inconstant blood flow
- Inappropriate administration of contrast media may mimic thrombus.

Modification to technique: Plain study can be obtained as a HRCT.

IV contrast: 60-100 ml based on indication.

CHEST, GENERAL

Indications: Suspected or known pulmonary, pleural or lymph node disease, including metastatic neoplasms, infection, traumatic lesions and focal diseases.

Advisable preliminary investigations: Chest radiography.

Patient preparation: Information about the procedure; restraint from food, but not fluid, is recommended, if intravenous contrast media are to be given.

Scan projection radiograph: Frontal from neck to upper abdomen.

Image criteria:
Visualization of:
- Entire thoracic wall
- Entire thoracic aorta and vena cava
- Entire heart
- Entire lung parenchyma
- Vessels after intravenous contrast media.

Patient position: Supine, arms above the head.

Volume of investigation: From lung apex to the base of the lungs.

Nominal slice thickness: 7-10 mm serial or preferably helical.

Inter-slice distance/pitch: Contiguous or a pitch = 1.0; or pitch up to 1.5 may be used for large lesions or detection of lymphadenopathy alone; even larger inter-slice distance/pitch may be applied in critically ill patients.

FOV: Adjusted to the largest thoracic diameter within the volume of investigation.

Gantry tilt: None.

X-ray tube voltage (kV): Standard.

Tube current and exposure time product (mAs): Should be as low as consistent with required image quality.

Reconstruction algorithm: Soft tissue/standard.

Window width: 300-600 HU (soft tissue), 800-1.600 HU (lung parenchyma).

Window level: 0-30 HU (soft tissue, unenhanced examination), 30-60 HU (soft tissue, enhanced examination), 500 to 700 HU (lung parenchyma).

Motion: Movement artifact deteriorates the image quality. This is prevented by a standard breath-hold technique; alternatively if this is not possible scan during quiet respiration.

Intravenous contrast media: May be used to characterize lesions or to distinguish them from vessels.

Pitfalls:
- Anatomical misregistration due to variation in the phase of respiration
- Focal atelectasis may obscure pathology
- Motion artifact due to cardiac pulsation or respiration.

Modification to technique:
- Prone position may be used to elucidate pleural lesions or focal spaces
- The examination may be confined to a specific area of interest
- 2 mm slices may be used for specific examination of hilar pathology and subtle pulmonary lesions.

CHEST, HRCT (HIGH RESOLUTION CT)

Indications: Detection and characterization of diffuse parenchymal lung disease including emphysema or bronchiectasis.

Advisable preliminary investigations: Chest radiography and respiratory function tests.

Patient preparation: Information about the procedure.

Scan projection radiograph: Frontal from neck to upper abdomen.

Image criteria:
Visualization of:
- Entire field of lung parenchyma.

Patient position: Supine, arms above the head.

Volume of investigation: From lung apex to the base of the lungs (survey) or corresponding to radiographically defined abnormality (localized disease).

Nominal slice thickness: 1-2 mm.

Inter-slice distance/pitch: 10-20 mm.

FOV: Adjusted to the minimum which will demonstrate the whole lung field.

Gantry tilt: None.

X-ray tube voltage (kV): High kV or standard.

Tube current and exposure time product (mAs): Should be as low as consistent with required image quality.

Reconstruction algorithm: High resolution.

Window width: 1000-1600 HU.

Window level: -400 to -700 HU.

Problems and pitfalls:
- Motion artifact due to dyspnea
- Atelectasis may obscure pathology.

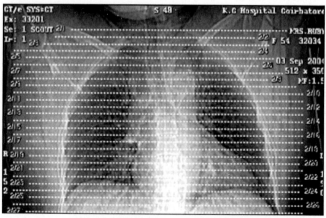

Fig. 5.6: Scan plan for HRCT chest

Modification to technique: Prone position may be used to elucidate dependent changes, especially small areas of atelectasis

- Examination in suspended expiration to detect air trapping
- Sections with smaller inter-slice distance for evaluation of very small areas of disease
- Sections with a cranio-caudal –25 to –30° gantry tilt for detection of bronchiectasis.

ABDOMEN, GENERAL

Indications: Inflammatory lesions, abscess, suspected or known structural alteration or space-occupying lesions of the abdomen and retroperitoneum, lesions of major vessels such as aneurysms and traumatic lesions, and as a guide to biopsy.

Advisable preliminary investigations: Ultrasonography.

Patient preparation: Information about the procedure; exclude high density contrast media from previous investigations; oral application of contrast media for the intestine; restraint from food, but not fluid, is recommended, if intravenous contrast media are to be given.

Scan projection radiograph: Frontal from lower chest to pelvis.

Image criteria:
Visualization of:
- Diaphragm
- Entire liver and spleen
- Retroperitoneal parenchymal organs (pancreas, kidneys).

- Abdominal aorta and the proximal part of the common iliac arteries
- Abdominal wall including all herniations
- Vessels after intravenous contrast media.

Patient position: Supine with arms at chest or head level.

Volume of investigation: From dome of the liver to the aortic bifurcation.

Nominal slice thickness: 7-10 mm; 4-5 mm for dedicated indications only (suspected small lesions), serial or preferably helical.

Inter-slice distance/pitch: Contiguous or a pitch = 1.0; in screening investigations, e.g. for traumatic lesions < 10 mm or a pitch up to 1.2-2.0.

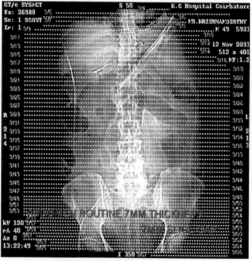

Fig. 5.7: Scan plan for abdomen

FOV: Adjusted to the largest abdominal diameter.

Gantry tilt: None.

X-ray tube voltage (kV): Standard.

Tube current and exposure time product (mAs): Should be as low as consistent with required image quality.

Reconstruction algorithm: Standard or soft tissue.

Window width: 150-600 HU, 2000-3000 HU (bone, if required).

Window level: 30-60 HU (enhanced examination), 0-30 HU (unenhanced examination), 400-600 HU (bone, if required).

Motion: Movement artifact deteriorates the image quality. This is prevented by a standard breath-hold technique; alternatively, if this is not possible scan during quiet respiration.

Intravenous contrast media: Useful for differentiating vessels and organ tissues from adjacent structures and to detect parenchymal lesions in solid organs.

Problems and pitfalls
- Non-contrasted parts of the intestine may mimic tumours
- The delineation of organs and structures may be poor in cachectic patients with reduced intra-abdominal and retroperitoneal fat.

Modification to technique: Helical CT which is beneficial for elimination of motion artifact can be used for demonstrating vascular pathologies may be combined with examination of the pelvis. CT colonograpy can be done were indicated.

IV contrast: 80-120 ml based on patient size and indication.

PELVIS

General Preparatory Steps

Indications: Disorders of the prostate, uterus or female gonads and suspected or known focal or diffuse structural disease of the pelvis, e.g. lymphomas.

Advisable preliminary investigations: Ultrasonography; endoscopy (for intraluminal pathology).

Patient preparation: Information about the procedure; exclude high density contrast media from previous investigations; administration of oral or rectal contrast media for bowel demarcation; vaginal contrast tampon in gynecological indications. Urinary bladder should not be empty; restraint from food, but not fluid, is recommended, if intravenous contrast media are to be given.

Scan projection radiograph: Frontal from iliac crest to proximal femur.

Image criteria:
Visualization of:
- Entire iliac bones
- Entire ischial bones
- Entire pubic symphysis
- Entire urinary bladder
- All peripelvic muscles
- Vessels after intravenous contrast media.

Patient position: Supine with arms at chest or head level.

Volume of investigation: From iliac crest to pelvic floor.

Nominal slice thickness: 7-10 mm; 4-5 mm if small lesions are suspected, serial or preferably helical CT.

Inter-slice distance/pitch: Contiguous or a pitch = 1.0; 4-5 mm or a pitch up to 1.2-1.5 may be used in screening examinations.

FOV: Adjusted to the maximum diameter of the pelvis.

Gantry tilt: None.

X-ray tube voltage (kV): Standard.

Tube current and exposure time product (mAs): Should be as low as consistent with required image quality.

Reconstruction algorithm: Soft tissue/standard or high resolution if bone evaluation is required.

Window width: 200-600 HU (soft tissues), 2000-3000 HU (bones).

Window level: 30-60 HU (enhanced examination), 0-30 HU (unenhanced examination), 400-600 HU (bones).

Protective shielding: Lead-shielding for the gonads.

Pitfalls:
- Delineation of organs and structures may be difficult in cachectic patients with reduced intra-abdominal and retroperitoneal fatty tissue
- Folds of the bowel wall or stool may mimic tumor
- Empty urinary bladder
- Contrast media "jets" from the ureters into the urinary bladder.

Modification to technique: Additional thinner slices to delineate small alterations
- Additional enteral contrast media may be needed to visualize the bowel
- Additional, iv contrast media with regard to the urinary bladder
- Filling of the urinary bladder by oral water intake.

OSSEOUS PELVIS

Indications: Evaluation or verification of pelvic ring and acetabular fractures, hip dislocation, bone tumours, degenerative, infectious, arthritic and osteonecrotic changes.

Advisable preliminary investigations: Always conventional radiography; MRI or ultrasonography may be alternative examinations without exposure to ionising radiation in non-traumatic disorders.

Patient preparation: Information about the procedure; restraint from food, but not fluid, is recommended, if intravenous contrast media are to be given.

Scan projection radiograph: Frontal from iliac crest to ischial tuberosity.

Image criteria:
Visualization of:
- Whole pelvic ring
- Hip(s) including the trochanter region
- Sacroiliac joints
- Pubic symphysis.

Patient position: Supine with arms at chest or head level.

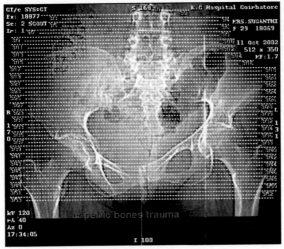

Fig. 5.8: Scanogram of pelvis

Volume of investigation: Tumour/fracture: from 1 cm above to 1 cm below; the diseased area; joint disorders: 1 cm above to 1 cm below the joint region.

Nominal slice thickness: 3-5 mm in the hip region; 3-10 mm outside the hip, serial or preferably helical.

Inter-slice distance/pitch: Contiguous or pitch = 1.0 in the hip region, < 5 mm or a pitch up to 1.2-1.5 outside the hip region.

FOV: Pelvis, hip or sacroiliac joint dimension (usually 15-40 cm).

Gantry tilt: Usually none, but cranial tilting should be used for examination of the sacroiliac joints to reduce radiation to the female gonads.

X-ray tube voltage (kV): Standard or high kV in large persons to avoid noise.

Tube current and exposure time product (mAs): Should be as low as consistent with required image quality.

Reconstruction algorithm: Soft tissue/standard or high resolution.

Window width: 1000-1500 HU (joints/bones), 200-600 HU (soft tissue).

Window level: 150-200 HU (joints/bones), 30-50 HU (soft tissue).

Protective shielding: Lead-shield for the gonads.

Problems and pitfalls: Artifact due to metallic objects such as prothesis.

Modification to technique: IV contrast media to delineate traumatic lesion of pelvic organs.

PROTOCOLS FOR COMMON CLINICAL INDICATION

Acute Abdomen

Injection rate	3 cc/sec
Contrast volume and type	80-100 ionic/nonionic
Area scanned	From diaphragm to symphysis pubis
Scan delay	25 sec
Length of spiral (time)	30-40 sec
Slice thickness	7 mm
Table speed/pitch	7 mm/sec

Reconstruction interval	As decided by the radiologist

Comment: 750 cc of oral contrast (3% gastroscan) is given in divided doses beginning approximately one hour prior to the study. Delayed scans may be useful in select cases. In cases of suspected pelvic abscess, rectal contrast may prove useful to define the position of the rectum and sigmoid colon.

Abdomen—Trauma

Injection rate	3 ml/sec
Contrast volume and type	135 ml of 60%
Area scanned	

1. Highest hemidiaphragm through kidneys
2. Below kidneys through ischial rami.

Scan delay	70 sec/additional 70 sec
Length of spiral (time)	30-40 sec/nonspiral
Slice thickness	5 mm
Table speed/pitch	1.5 pitch/5 mm increments
Reconstruction interval	5 mm
3D technique used	None

Comment:
- Oral contrast is routinely given (water-soluble agent).
- Rectal contrast is given when colon injury is suspected.

Abdomen—Livermass

Specific anatomic region	Liver
Application	Differential diagnosis of liver masses
Injection rate	2.5-3 ml/sec
Contrast volume and type	80-120 ml of ionic/nonionic contrast
Area scanned	Entire liver
Scan delay	25 sec arterial/60 sec venous
Length of spiral (time)	Approx 30 sec
Slice thickness	5 mm
Table speed/pitch	Pitch 1-1.5
Reconstruction interval	3 mm intervals
3D technique used	None

Suspected Hemangioma

Specific anatomic region	Liver
Application	Suspected hemangioma
Injection rate	2-3 ml/sec
Contrast volume and type	100 ml of non ionic
Area scanned	Sequential images over suspected lesion
Scan delay	25 sec to initial scan
Length of spiral (time)	Not needed
Slice thickness	5 mm
Table speed/pitch	N/A
Reconstruction interval	N/A
3D technique used	N/A

Comment: Scans are obtained at 30 sec intervals until 5 min, then at 10 min to note the classic peripheral enhancement and fill in for these tumors.

PANCREAS

Pancreatitis

Injection rate	2-3 ml/sec
Contrast volume and type	80-100 nonionic
Area scanned	From diaphragm to iliac crest
Scan delay	25 sec
Length of spiral (time)	30-40 sec
Slice thickness	5 mm
Table speed/pitch	5-7 mm/sec
Reconstruction interval	2-3 mm as needed
3D technique used	Volume rendering

Pancreatic Mass

Injection rate	3.5 ml/sec
Contrast volume and type	75–100 cc of nonionic contrast
Area scanned	Diaphragm to iliac crest Liver and pancreas in arterial-phase study.
Scan delay	20 sec for arterial phase/60 sec for venous phase
Length of spiral (time)	25 sec
Slice thickness	3 mm
Table speed/pitch	4.5 mm/sec or a pitch of 1.5
Reconstruction interval	1.3 mm
3D technique used	MIP to denote the vascular relationship. Volume rendering can also be used

Endocrine Tumours of Pancreas

Injection rate	3-4 ml/sec
Contrast volume and type	100-120 ml of nonionic contrast
Area scanned	Area of pancreas first defined on contrast scan
Scan delay	Arterial phase determined by test bolus injection
Length of spiral (time)	20 sec
Slice thickness	5 mm
Table speed/pitch	5 mm/sec or a pitch of 1
Reconstruction interval	2 mm
3D technique used	None

Comment: The arterial phase is classically best for vascular tumors like an islet cell tumor. It is best to opacify c loop with water so that the enhancement is not obscured.

R/O Renal or Ureteral Calculus

Application	R/O renal or ureteral calculus
Injection rate	No contrast used
Contrast volume and type	N/A
Area scanned	From midportion T-12 to midportion of symphysis
Scan delay	None
Length of spiral (time)	Up to 40 sec

Slice thickness	3 mm
Table speed/pitch	6 mm/sec
Reconstruction interval	3 mm
3D technique used	None usually

Comment: Reformatting of data into oblique planes may better define the location of a stone in difficult cases.

Staging Renal Mass

Injection rate	3 ml/sec
Contrast volume and type	120 ml of Omnipaque-350
Area scanned	
Arterial phase (AP)	2 cm above and below kidney.
Delayed phase (DP)	From diaphragm to symphysis
Scan delay	30 sec, 70 sec (dual spiral)
Length of spiral (time)	Usually 30 sec for arterial and 40 sec for delayed phase
Slice thickness	3 mm (AP) 5 mm (DP)
Table speed/pitch	5 mm/ sec (AP), 8 mm/ sec (DP)
Reconstruction interval	3 mm (AP), 5 mm (DP)
3D technique used	Volume rendering on arterial phase.

Evaluate Suspected Renal Artery Stenosis

Injection rate	3 cc/sec
Contrast volume and type	100-120 cc

Area scanned	Through regions of renal arteries
Scan delay	25-30 sec
Length of spiral (time)	20-30 sec each
Slice thickness	2-3 mm
Table speed/pitch	4-6 mm/sec
Reconstruction interval	1 mm
3D technique used	Volume rendering and MIP

Comment: Non-contrast CTs are first obtained to localize the renal arteries for the CT angiogram. This allows a smaller scan volume which is critical with SDCT and the use of 1-2 mm collimation. 3D with VRT is accurate to quantify stenosis.

Renal Donor Evaluation

Injection rate	3.5 ml/sec (mean)
Contrast volume and type	80-100 ml nonionic contrast
Area scanned	Entire kidneys
Scan delay	20 sec
Length of spiral (time)	Approx 30 sec
Slice thickness	3 mm
Table speed/pitch	3-5 mm
Reconstruction interval	2 mm
3D technique used	MIP

Comment: 15 minutes after contrast injection, conventional radiographs (AP, obliques) can be obtained if the urologists desires so.

Stomach: Gastric Mass

Injection rate	2-3 ml/sec
Contrast volume and rype	80-100 ml of nonionic contrast
Area scanned	From diaphragm to top of iliac crest
Scan delay	24 sec
Length of spiral (time)	Up to 30-40 sec
Slice thickness	3 mm
Table speed/pitch	5 mm/sec
Reconstruction interval	2-3 mm

Comment: Distension of the stomach with 750 cc of 3% gastrograffin or 750-1000 cc of water. This allows better evaluation of the gastric wall and definition of tumors, etc.

Colon: Suspected Diverticulitis

Injection rate	3 cc/sec
Contrast volume and type	80-100
Area scanned	From diaphragm to symphysis
Scan delay	50 sec
Length of spiral (time)	32-40 sec
Slice thickness	5 mm
Table speed/pitch	8 mm/sec
Reconstruction interval	5 mm
3D technique used	None

Comment: A focused exam of the colon requires P.O. contrast 90-120 minutes before the study. If necessary, rectal contrast may be given.

Appendix, Cecum: R/O Appendicitis

Injection rate	80-100 ml nonionic IV contrast.
Contrast volume and type	750 ml oral contrast; 300-800 ml rectal contrast
Area scanned	From L2 level
Scan delay	40 min delay between oral contrast and CT scan. 25 seconds delay for IV contrast
Length of spiral (time)	30 sec
Slice thickness	5 mm
Table speed/pitch	5 mm/sec or a pitch of 1
Reconstruction interval	5 mm
3D technique used	If needed VR may be used

Pelvic

Application	Cervical cancer, bladder cancer
Injection rate	3 ml/sec
Contrast volume and type	110-120 ml of non ionic
Area scanned	From symphysis pubis through iliac crest followed by scans through the diaphragm
Scan delay	25 sec
Length of spiral (time)	30 sec followed by a second spiral to screen the abdomen

Slice thickness	3-5 mm for pelvis, 7 mm for the abdominal screening.
Table speed/pitch	3-5 mm/sec
Reconstruction interval	3-5 mm
3D technique used	None routinely needed

Ovarian Mass/Cancer

Injection rate	2 cc/sec
Contrast volume and type	80-100 of nonionic
Area scanned	Diaphragm through symphysis pubis
Scan delay	50 sec
Length of spiral (time)	30-40 sec
Slice thickness	5 mm
Table speed/pitch	7 mm
Reconstruction interval	3 mm

Comment:
- Delayed scans through the pelvis at 5 minutes post-injection allow adequate bladder opacification
- Rectal contrast may be helpful for defining spread of tumor in the pelvis.

Fistula to Bladder

Injection rate	None used
Contrast volume and type	None used
Area scanned	From iliac crest to symphysis pubis
Scan delay	None
Length of spiral (time)	30 sec
Slice thickness	5 mm

Table speed/pitch	5 mm/sec
Reconstruction interval	5 mm
3D technique used	MPR

Comment: Contrast is given via rectum and reflux in to urinary bladder.

Musculoskeletal Shoulder: Trauma to Shoulder Joint

Injection rate	N/A
Contrast volume and type	N/A
Area scanned	From just above acromioclavicular joint through scapular tip
Scan delay	None
Length of spiral (time)	40 sec
Slice thickness	3 mm
Table speed/pitch	3-5 mm/sec

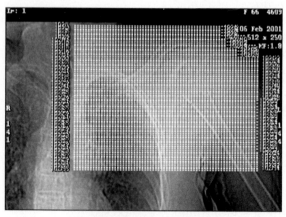

Fig. 5.9: Scan plan for shoulder

| Reconstruction interval | 2 mm |
| 3D technique used | Volume rendering and multiplanar obliques |

Comment: The technique can be modified if only the humeral head is injured. In cases with complex trauma *IV contrast* may be used to exclude a vascular injury to the mediastinum. The protocol used would use 120 ml of contrast injected at 3 ml/sec with a 30 sec delay.

Specific Anatomic Region Wrist

Application	1.R/O fracture, R/O Fx/dislocation
Injection rate	N/A
Contrast volume and type	N/A
Area scanned	Entire wrist
Scan delay	None
Length of spiral (time)	15-25 sec
Slice thickness	2 mm
Table speed/pitch	2-3 mm
Reconstruction interval	1-2 mm
3D technique used	Volume rendering

Comment: The best plane to scan is with the patient's arm in the scanner parallel to the X-ray beam.

Specific Anatomic Region Acetabulum/Pelvis

Application	Evaluate suspected fracture
Injection rate	N/A
Contrast volume and type	N/A
Area scanned	From iliac crest through ischium

Scan delay	None
Length of spiral (time)	40 sec
Slice thickness	3 mm
Table speed/pitch	1.6 pitch
Reconstruction interval	2 mm
3D technique used	Volume rendering

Comment: IV contrast can be used to create vascular maps to exclude vascular injury. In these cases a delay of 30 sec till scanning is ideal. A CT cystogram may also be useful in these cases.

Knee: Trauma

Injection rate	None
Contrast volume and type	None
Area scanned	Tibial plateau
Scan delay	None
Length of spiral (time)	30-40 sec
Slice thickness	2 mm
Table speed/pitch	2 mm/sec
Reconstruction interval	1 mm
3D technique used	Vr, mpvr.

Ankle: Evaluate Suspected Fracture

Application	Evaluate suspected fracture
Injection rate	N/A
Contrast volume and type	N/A
Area scanned	Several cm above the talotibial joint through the midfoot
Scan delay	None
Length of spiral (time)	30-40 sec

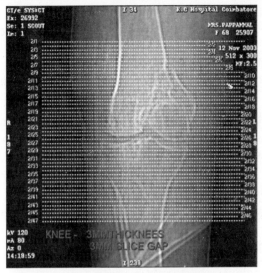

Fig. 5.10: Scan plan for knee

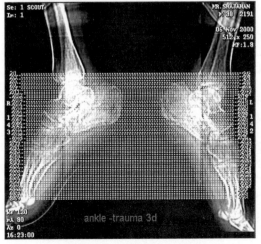

Fig. 5.11: Scan plan for ankle

Slice thickness	3 mm
Table speed/pitch	Usually 3 mm/sec or a pitch of 1
Reconstruction interval	1 or 3 mm
3D technique used	Volume rendering and MPR

Comment: This technique relies on a single CT acquisition in a plane parallel to the foot with MPR and 3D reconstructions done to provide all views.

Cervical Spine: Trauma—Extent of Injury

Application	Trauma—extent of injury
Injection rate	N/A
Contrast volume and type	None used
Area Scanned	From craniocervical junction to the top of T-1
Scan delay	None
Length of spiral (time)	Not defined
Slice thickness	3 mm
Table speed/pitch	1.5 pitch
Reconstruction interval	1 mm
3D technique used	? shaded surface ? MPR

Comments: IV contrast is given if vascular injury is also suspected.

Orbit: Trauma

Injection rate	N/A
Contrast volume and type	None used

Area scanned	Coronal—from front of eyelids to behind the optic canals. Axial—through orbits.
Scan delay	None
Length of spiral (time)	Not defined
Slice thickness	Coronal: 1 mm Axial: 1 mm
Table speed/pitch	Coronal: 1.5 mm/sec Axial: 1 mm
Reconstruction interval	Coronal: 1 mm Axial: 1 mm
3D technique used	Shaded surface rendering

Comments:
1. This protocol is also used for foreign body localization.
2. Images are filmed at both soft tissue and bone windows.

Facial Region: Trauma

Injection rate	N/A
Contrast volume and type	None used
Area scanned	Coronal—from front of nasal bone to behind sphenoid sinuses. Axial—from below maxillae to above frontal sinuses.
Scan delay	None
Length of spiral (time)	Not defined
Slice thickness	Coronal: 3 mm Axial: 3 mm

Table speed/pitch	Coronal: 4.5 mm/sec
	Axial: 4.5 mm/sec
Reconstruction interval	Coronal: 3 mm or 1
	Axial: 3 mm or 1
3D technique used	Shaded surface (SSD)

Comments:
1. Scanning is done in both coronal and axial plane.
2. Data is reconstructed at 1 mm interval when MPR or 3D is done.

Neck—Adenopathy

Injection rate	1 ml/sec
Contrast volume and type	100 ml of Omnipaque-300
Area scanned	Cervical region
Scan delay	30 sec
Length of spiral (time)	40 sec

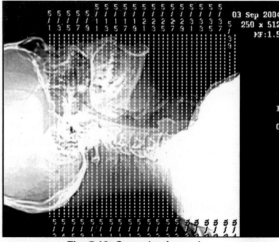

Fig. 5.12: Scan plan for neck

Slice thickness	5 mm
Table speed/pitch	5 mm/sec
Reconstruction interval	5 mm
3D technique used	None used

Comment:
1. With spiral CT this can easily be combined with an examination of the chest.
2. I think this flow rate is just too low for a good study. A flow rate of 2-2.5 ml/sec is ideal.

Anatomic Region: Pulmonary Artery

Application	R/O pulmonary embolism
Injection rate	3 ml/sec
Contrast volume and type	80-120 ml
Area scanned	Level of just above aortic arch through lung bases
Scan delay	25 sec
Length of spiral (time)	30-35 sec
Slice thickness	3 mm
Table speed/pitch	5 mm/ sec
Reconstruction interval	2 mm
3D technique used	Volume rendering / MIP/ MPR. This protocol is followed by screening of leg and pelvic veins.

Thoracic Aorta: R/O Dissection

Specific anatomic region	Thoracic aorta
Application	R/O dissection

Chapter 6

Post Processing Techniques

MULTIPLANAR RECONSTRUCTION (MPR)

The 3D nature of volume images acquired using helical CT allows for simple and efficient computation of images that lie along the non-acquired orthogonal orientations of the volume. It is a very fast and inter-active algorithm, suitable to represent several arbitrary planes at once. Implementations of multiplanar reconstruction techniques (MPR) on modern computers allow interactive generation and display of these images in real-time on multipanal displays. From the early days of CT, MPR is being used as a tool to provide arbitrary planes from transaxial slices. MPR, however, is not considered to be a true 3D representation and the image quality is limited by the z-resolution of the CT data set. Therefore, MPR have not been used much in conventional CT since spatial resolution along the z-axis used to be poor and stair step artifacts were common. With the advent of MDCT with the possi-bility of isotropic data sets, artifacts can be eliminated but image quality still depends on acquisition para-meters. Using thin collimation, excellent results are obtained.

Generally, MPR are helpful whenever pathology cannot be accurately assessed on axial images alone. Most situations involve pathologic interfaces that are oriented parallel to the axial plane or structures that cannot be displayed in their entirety since they run through a number of slices. In these cases, problem-oriented imaging planes can be generated using MPR. MPR is the fastest reconstruction method and almost everywhere available.

MPR also serve as an important communication tool with the referring physicians and play a major role in orthopedic and trauma therapy planning.

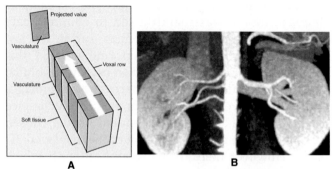

Figs 6.1A and B: Diagram showing the basis of MPR

SURFACE RENDERING [SHADED SURFACE DISPLAY (SSD)]

The "Marching Cubes" algorithm must be considered the hallmark of surface rendering. Prior to applying the algorithm, the user specifies a threshold value and by doing so selects the objects to be rendered.

This specification has vast ramifications regarding the quality and accuracy of the object depiction. The threshold needs to be adapted to the individual application under consideration, e.g. bone, soft tissue.

Once the threshold has been determined, the surface rendering algorithm loops on each successive group of four adjacent data slices. The slices are read into memory and each cell is scanned to determine whether its corner values straddle the threshold value. Non-straddling cells are discarded. Cells that do straddle the threshold are examined more closely. The eight corners of the cube are valued "1" if their signal exceeds the threshold and "0" if it does not. They form an eight bitbyte,

Surface rendering, also called shades surface displays (SSD), was mainly used to communicate findings to the referring physicians during the last decade. Using larger data sets performing MDCT, this visualization role will be overtaken by newer volume rendering techniques. While surface rendering images are very intuitive, they are also prone to artifacts since image quality is strongly dependent on the chosen threshold range for the definition of the displayed 3D object. However, there are many applications in which radiology truly benefits from SSD. These include all procedures for surgical planning and 3D renderings of complex acetabular fractures, facial fractures, orthopedic deformities, CT angiography of the thoracic aorta and preoperative planning for interventional endovascular procedures. The classification of

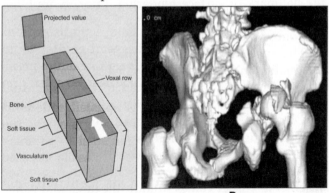

Figs 6.2A and B: Diagram showing SSD

acetabular fractures is markedly simplified with 3D reconstructions

Complex procedures in craniofacial surgery also benefit from surface rendering

VOLUME RENDERING (VR)

Volume rendering is the representation, visualization, and manipulation of objects represented as sampled data in three or more dimensions. Volume rendering displays visual images directly from volume data, enabling the viewer to fully reveal the internal structure of 3D data. Rather than editing a single scan, volume rendering interpolates the entire data set. Speaking of image post processing, volume rendering is one of the most important software techniques

With standard orthographic imaging, such as shaded surface display or MIP, changing position can cause distortions in the image. With perspective

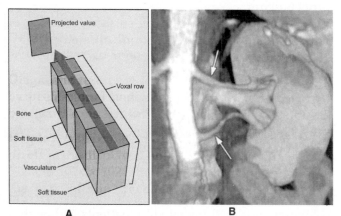

A   B

Figs 6.3A and B: Diagrams showing the basis of volume rendering

volume rendering, there is no distortion. Perspective volume rendering requires a data set that permits 3D imaging, which basically means one with thin collimation.

The rendering is performed by a software technique that assigns both opacity and color to each voxel in the data set.

Once the volume rendering display has been compiled, the opacity can be suppressed in order to examine different tissues.

VIRTUAL ENDOSCOPY (VE)

Virtual endoscopy (VE) describes a new method of diagnosis, using computer processing of 3D image data sets (such as from spiral or multidetector CT scans) to provide simulated visualizations of patient—specific organs similar or equivalent to those produced by standard endoscopic procedures, such as colonoscopy, bronchoscopy.

VE can be performed using surface rendering or volume rendering based either on volumetric CT.

VIRTUAL COLONOSCOPY

Virtual colonoscopy techniques have been introduced as potential methods for colorectal screening and preoperative staging, and combine volumetric imaging based on CT with sophisticated image processing.

This technique is particularly attractive due to the increased potential for patient compliance.

Screening for colorectal cancer with virtual colonoscopy is well tolerated by patients, although it does involve a cleansing preparation for the colon. The procedure is safe, and the 3D images are quite compelling and allow for a number of unique abilities, such as separating out polyps from nodular folds by virtually splitting the colon open.

The data sets for virtual colonoscopy are acquired using 4 × 1 mm slice collimation, slice thickness 1.25 mm, data reconstruction interval 1 mm and a pitch of 6.

Radiologists using this technology must also look carefully to see whether there is any air within a filling defect of the colon. Even on the endoscopic views, fecal residue can look relatively rounded, and so endoscopic views alone will not suffice: radiologists must refer back to the axial source images.

VIRTUAL BRONCHOSCOPY

Virtual bronchoscopy is emerging as a useful approach for assessment of three dimensional reconstructed airways.

1. Preprocessing of image data, which involves extracting objects of interest, defining paths through major airways, and preparing the extracted objects for 3D rendering; and interactive image.

2. Assessment, which involves use of graphics-based software tools such as surface-rendered views, projection images, virtual endoscopic views, oblique section images, measurement data and cross-sectional views. Although a virtual bronchoscope offers a unique opportunity for exploration and quantitation, it cannot replace a real bronchoscope.

Virtual endoscopy reproduces real endoscopic images but cannot provide information on the aspect of the mucosa or biopsy specimens. It offers possible applications for preparing, guiding and controlling interventional fibroscopy procedures.

However, virtual bronchoscopy based on MSCT data permits to investigate peripheral bronchi far beyond those that can be examined by a physical bronchoscope. Indications for virtual bronchoscopy include evaluation of bronchial anastomosis following lung transplantation, evaluation of abnormalities of the central airways after intubation, tracheotomy or irradiation of the neck, bronchial stenosis in Wegener granulomatosis, and airway reconstruction after tumor resection functional imaging of the tracheobronchial tree is also possible by acquiring a scan in inspiration as well as in expiration. Furthermore, the MDCT data can be used to generate an interactive 3D virtual bronchoscopic approach for preoperative endotracheal stent planning.

Biopsy Planning

In the past, if a patient had a tumor in the chest, abdomen, or pelvis, surgery was required in order to make a definite diagnosis and determine the specific type of tumor before appropriate therapy could be implemented. This approach is certainly acceptable if the patient would require surgery anyway in order to treat the tumor. However, many patients have types of tumors in which surgery is not indicated (frequently patients with metastatic disease), and other patients are not surgical candidates because of additional medical conditions. CT guided, percutaneous (i.e. through the skin) needle biopsy has developed into the frequently used alternative to open surgical exploration and biopsy.

Indications and Contraindications

Almost any organ or structure in the body can be biopsied percutaneously under CT guidance. This includes the lungs, mediastinum, liver, kidneys, adrenal glands, pancreas, retroperitoneum, and pelvis. The spleen is seldom biopsied because it is a highly vascular organ and the risk of severe post-biopsy hemorrhage is significant. Most biopsies are performed to confirm that a mass is malignant, and to determine the specific type of tumor so that appropriate therapy can be started. Some biopsies are performed to evaluate the type and severity of benign disease (e.g. liver biopsy for hepatitis, renal biopsy for glomerulo-nephritis).

Relative contraindications to CT guided biopsy include:
- Patients with uncorrectable bleeding disorders. The risk of post-biopsy hemorrhage is too high.
- Lesions in which a safe biopsy path cannot be found. This includes deep tumors which the needle could only reach by traversing large blood vessels (in the chest, abdomen, or pelvis), bowel (in the abdomen or pelvis), or other vital organs (e.g. the spleen, heart, aorta).
- Lesions which will be surgically resected regardless of the biopsy result. This applies to many solitary lung and kidney masses.

- Suspected types of lesions in which the risk of life-threatening post-biopsy complications is high. This includes pulmonary arteriovenous malformation, cavernous hemangioma or echinococcal cyst of the liver.
- Patients who cannot cooperate with the exam.

Risks

CT guided biopsy is a relatively safe procedure. The risks are almost always less than surgical biopsy, which would be the most common alternative. The recovery time is considerably less than surgery.

Risks of CT guided biopsy depend somewhat on the site being biopsied. These risks include:

- Bleeding: Most patients have evaluation of their blood clotting status prior to biopsy. Although rare, bleeding can be life-threatening and can require surgery to correct.
- Infection: Infection can develop anytime a needle pierces the skin. However, sterile technique is used during the biopsy and this is a very rare complication.
- Pneumothorax: A reported complication in up to 25% of lung biopsies (although only a few of these patients require a chest tube). Also a risk during biopsies in the upper abdomen (usually liver and adrenal).
- Damage to adjacent organs: Although CT can accurately locate the lesion, the biopsy is not performed under real time imaging. Patient movement and variation in breathing can alter the relationship of the lesion and adjacent organs, including bowel and vascular structures.

Technique

The technique will vary based on the lesion being biopsied and any limitations of the patient. A generalized sequence is as follows:

- The patient can lie on the CT table on their back, on their stomach, or on either side, depending on the needle path planned. Although systemic anesthesia is usually not required, some patients will receive intravenous sedation and/or pain relief.
- Limited CT scanning is performed, and the lesion is located. The safest and easiest path for the needle is planned.
- The overlying skin is cleaned and draped in a sterile manner. The skin and underlying tissue is anesthetized. Once the depth and angulation of the needle is determined from the CT images, the needle is placed through the skin into the body.
- Additional CT images are obtained to confirm that the tip of the needle lies in the lesion. Adjustments to the needle position are made as necessary.
- When the tip of the needle is shown to lie in the proper position, the biopsy is obtained. Different types of needles are available. Some are for aspiration (obtains scattered cells from the lesion), and others are cutting needles which obtain a small core of tissue.
- A preliminary evaluation of the specimen is frequently performed by the pathologist. If there is sufficient tissue for diagnosis, the procedure is terminated. If not, additional biopsies will be obtained.

- The patient is observed either in the department or in a short-stay nursing unit for 2 to 4 hours, and then sent home. If there are no complications, admission to the hospital is seldom required.

BIOPSY SCAN

Biopsy Scan 1

Function

The biopsy Rx feature allows you to easily repeat the scan location during the biopsy procedures. Example given below is from a CT/E scanner from Ge.

Biopsy Rx Prescription

1. Biopsy Rx can be accessed through the (Biopsy Rx) icon on the righ side of axial/helical prescription screen.
2. The following screen appears upon the selection of (biopsy Rx).

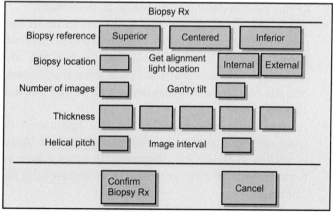

Fig. 6.4: Schematic representation of planning biopsy

Biopsy Scan 2

1. In order to determine the reference centering in a biopsy scan, select (superior), (centered) or (inferior) at biopsy reference field.
   - Superior means scanning from the landmark toward patient's head
   - Centered means scanning around the landmark.
   - Inferior means scanning from the landmark toward patient's feet
2. When the internal light is used, select (internal) or when the external light is used select (external) at Get Alignment Light Location Field.
3. Enter the following parameters:
   - Number of images
   - Gantry tilt
   - Thickness
   - Helical pitch
   - Image interval
4. Click on the (confirm biopsy Rx) button.
5. Press (move to scan) button when it lights up. Then, press (start scan) to start the biopsy scans.

Chapter 7

Contrast Issues

CT contrast agents, sometimes referred to as "dyes" are used to highlight specific areas so that the organs, blood vessels, or tissues are more visible. By increasing the visibility of all surfaces of the organ or tissue being studied, they can help the radiologist determine the presence and extent of disease or injury.

Contrast agents are available in several different forms, but in general a CT contrast agent is a pharmaceutical substance. Some of the more common contrast agents used are:

- Iodine
- Barium
- Barium sulfate
- Gastrografin

Contrast agents for CT examinations are administered in four different ways:

- Intravenous injection
- Oral administration
- Rectal administration
- Inhalation—This is a relatively uncommon procedure in which xenon gas is inhaled for a highly specialized form of lung or brain imaging. The technique, xenon CT, is only available at a small number of locations worldwide and is used only for rare cases.

INTRAVENOUS CONTRAST

Intravenous contrast is used to highlight blood vessels and to enhance the structure of organs like the brain, spine, liver, and kidney. The contrast agent (usually an iodine compound) is clear, with a water-like consistency. Typically the contrast is contained in a special injector, which injects the contrast through a small needle taped in place (usually on the back of the hand) during a specific period in the CT exam.

Once the contrast is injected into the bloodstream, it circulates throughout the body. The CT's X-ray beam is weakened as it passes through the blood vessels and organs that have "taken up" the contrast. These structures are enhanced by this process and show up as white areas on the CT images. When the test is finished, the kidneys and liver quickly eliminate the contrast from the body.

Iodinated Contrast Agents

Is Iodine a Safe Contrast Agent?

Iodine is considered to be a safe contrast agent. It has been used for many years without serious side effects. Because iodine contrast increases the visibility of target tissues on the images, the benefits are considered to outweigh the risks. The most common side effect of iodine is a warm or "flushed" sensation during the actual injection of the iodine, followed sometimes by a metallic taste in the mouth that usually lasts for less than a minute. No treatment is necessary for this sensation, if experienced.

Another mild reaction is itching over various parts of the body. This reaction lasts from several minutes to a few hours after the injection. When this reaction occurs, medication is usually administered to counteract the itching.

More serious allergic reactions, while uncommon, include difficulty breathing and swelling of the throat or other parts of the body. These reactions, if experienced, are treated immediately.

Newer forms of contrast help to reduce the risk of an allergic reaction. If you have had an allergic reaction to iodine or a contrast agent in the past, the physician may recommend on of these newer agents.

In some cases, CT can still provide valuable diagnostic information without the administration of a contrast agent, so the radiologist or a trained technologist may decide this is the best course of action.

ORAL CT CONTRAST

Oral contrast is used to highlight gastrointestinal (GI) organs in the abdomen and pelvis. If oral contrast will be used during an examination, the patient will be asked to fast for several hours before administration.

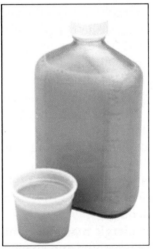

Fig. 7.1: Oral contrast agent

Two types of oral contrast are used:

Barium sulfate, the most common oral contrast agent, resembles a milkshake in appearance and consistency. The compound, available in various flavors, is prepared by mixing with water.

Gastrografin is a yellowish, water-based drink mixed with iodine. It can have a bitter taste.

When oral contrast has been requested by the doctor, patients usually drink about 1,000 to 1,500 cc over a one hour period.

After the contrast is swallowed, it travels to the stomach and gastrointestinal tract. Like intravenous iodine, barium and gastrografin weaken X-rays. On CT images, the organs that have "taken up" the contrast appear as highlighted white areas.

Is Oral Contrast Safe?

In general, both barium and gastrografin contrast are safe and pass uneventfully through the gastrointestinal tract. Minor and temporary side effects, such as constipation, may occur.

RECTAL CT CONTRAST

Rectal contrast is used when enhanced images of the large intestine and other lower GI organs are required. The same types of contrast used for oral contrast are used for rectal contrast, but in different concentrations.

Rectal CT contrast is usually administered by enema. When the contrast is administered, the patient may experience mild discomfort, coolness, and a sense of fullness. After the CT is complete, the contrast is drained and the patient may go to the bathroom.

The preparation for rectal contrast is similar to oral contrast, in that the patient should be fasting for several hours before the test. In addition, the patient will be required to use a Fleets Enema to cleanse the colon; it is usually used the night before the examination.

Is Rectal Contrast Safe?

Rectal contrast is considered to be safe and passes through the gastrointestinal tract uneventfully. Minor and temporary side effects, such as constipation, can occur.

Guidelines for IV Contrast Agent Reactions

Q. Radiographic contrast media adverse reactions?
Iodinated contrast media is routinely administered for many radiological procedures like CT, IVP or angiography. Due to the higher absorption of X-ray beams by the iodinated contrast, both normal and abnormal structures are better seen. However, because of the risks of adverse reaction to contrast administration in some patients, judicious use of these agents is required. The following are frequently asked questions about contrast media and contrast reactions.

Q. How frequently do allergic contrast reactions occur?
It is estimated that the overall frequency of adverse reactions is 5 to 10 percent. Most of these are very mild and may consist of only a few hives. However, in one of every 1,000 to 2,000 examinations, a moderate or severe reaction can occur. The risk of death from a

contrast agent is estimated to be 0.3 to 2.6 per 100,000 uses (comparable in magnitude to the risk of death from receiving a dose of penicillin).

Q. What types of allergic contrast reactions are seen?
Contrast reactions are classified as mild, moderate, or severe. Mild reactions include mild nausea and vomiting, mild urticaria and pruritus, and mild diaphoresis. Moderate reactions would include more severe presentations of the above symptoms, facial and laryngeal edema or mild bronchospasm. Severe reactions may include hypotensive shock, cardiac or respiratory arrest, pulmonary edema, loss of consciousness, convulsions, and severe laryngeal or bronchial spasm.

Q. How are these contrast reactions treated?
All contrast examinations are performed in the presence of a physician, usually a radiologist, the technician must be ready to initiate treatment of any reaction (Keep a guidelines for the treatment of these reactions in the CT gantry room). Most reactions are mild and require no treatment; outpatients are usually observed for 30 minutes for worsening of symptoms. In most cases, these mild symptoms are self-limiting and will resolve within this time with minimal or no treatment.

Q. What can be done if a patient with a history of contrast reaction needs another contrast exam?
This depends on the nature and severity of the prior reaction. If the prior reaction was mild, selection of a low-osmolar contrast agent ("non-ionic") and/or pretreatment with 25 to 50 mg of diphenhydramine

(avil) prior to the examination may be all that is needed. If the prior reaction was moderate or severe, a radiologist should be consulted to see if there is an alternative diagnostic imaging strategy (e.g. ultrasound or MRI) that avoids iodinated contrast exposure. Of note, gadolinium based MRI contrast agents have a different formulation from iodinated radiographic contrast media, and there is no known cross sensitivity between these two types of contrast.

If a contrast examination is still felt necessary, premedication with corticosteroids should be performed and low osmolar contrast selected. Two accepted protocols for corticosteroid administration in this setting include 50 mg of prednisone peroral. 12, 6, and 1 hour prior to the examination, or 32 mg of peroral solumedrol 12 and 2 hours prior to the exam. Fifty mg of diphenhydramine at bedtime the evening prior and 1 hour prior to the procedure is usually also administered. The equivalent IV dose of solumedrol can be substituted if the patient is unable to tolerate peroral administration.

Q. Are low-osmolar contrast media safer?

Low-osmolar contrast media (LOCM) are associated with less patient discomfort during administration. However, the risk of death from contrast reaction is felt to be mostly unchanged from that of high-osmolar contrast media (HOCM). The risk of very severe reactions is decreased with low osmolality contrast but the amount of risk reduction in patients not at high-risk for a reaction is very low. For the patient with no known risk factors for contrast reaction, HOCM are felt to be relatively safe.

Q. Why are LOCM not used routinely on all contrast examinations?

Low osmolality contrast agents are about 10 times more expensive than high osmolality agents. All outpatients who will undergo a contrast examination are screened by the radiologic technologist for risk factors including prior reaction, history of severe allergy to any medication, active asthma, current severe cardiac disease, history of sickle cell disease or multiple myeloma, and increased risk of aspiration. The radiologist then selects the dose and type of contrast media after reviewing this information. Formalize a protocol for the use of LOCM, patients can also be offered the choice by providing them with pamphlets detailing the contrast study.

Q. Do low osmolality contrast media have a lower incidence of associated nephrotoxicity?

Patients with insulin-dependent diabetes, volume depletion, and baseline renal dysfunction are a higher risk for contrast induced acute tubular necrosis or transient renal dysfunction. A few studies have suggested a slight benefit to use of LOCM in this setting. Contrast administration in patients with rising creatinine or stable creatine greater than 2.5 mg/dl is not recommended. LOCM is also often used in the patients with end-stage renal disease, not because of concerns of nephrotoxicity but due to the possible hemodynamic effects of an osmotic load in these patients that may also commonly have cardiac disease.

With the availability of new iso-osmolar contrast more at risk patients can be taken up for contrast studies in consultation with the nephrologist.

Virtual endoscopy reproduces real endoscopic images but cannot provide information on the aspect of the mucosa or biopsy specimens. It offers possible applications for preparing, guiding and controlling interventional fibroscopy procedures.

However, virtual bronchoscopy based on MSCT data permits to investigate peripheral bronchi far beyond those that can be examined by a physical bronchoscope. Indications for virtual bronchoscopy include evaluation of bronchial anastomosis following lung transplantation, evaluation of abnormalities of the central airways after intubation, tracheotomy or irradiation of the neck, bronchial stenosis in Wegener granulomatosis, and airway reconstruction after tumor resection functional imaging of the tracheobronchial tree is also possible by acquiring a scan in inspiration as well as in expiration. Furthermore, the MDCT data can be used to generate an interactive 3D virtual bronchoscopic approach for preoperative endotracheal stent planning.

Biopsy Planning

In the past, if a patient had a tumor in the chest, abdomen, or pelvis, surgery was required in order to make a definite diagnosis and determine the specific type of tumor before appropriate therapy could be implemented. This approach is certainly acceptable if the patient would require surgery anyway in order to treat the tumor. However, many patients have types of tumors in which surgery is not indicated (frequently patients with metastatic disease), and other patients are not surgical candidates because of additional medical conditions. CT guided, percutaneous (i.e. through the skin) needle biopsy has developed into the frequently used alternative to open surgical exploration and biopsy.

Indications and Contraindications

Almost any organ or structure in the body can be biopsied percutaneously under CT guidance. This includes the lungs, mediastinum, liver, kidneys, adrenal glands, pancreas, retroperitoneum, and pelvis. The spleen is seldom biopsied because it is a highly vascular organ and the risk of severe post-biopsy hemorrhage is significant. Most biopsies are performed to confirm that a mass is malignant, and to determine the specific type of tumor so that appropriate therapy can be started. Some biopsies are performed to evaluate the type and severity of benign disease (e.g. liver biopsy for hepatitis, renal biopsy for glomerulo-nephritis).

Relative contraindications to CT guided biopsy include:

- Patients with uncorrectable bleeding disorders. The risk of post-biopsy hemorrhage is too high.
- Lesions in which a safe biopsy path cannot be found. This includes deep tumors which the needle could only reach by traversing large blood vessels (in the chest, abdomen, or pelvis), bowel (in the abdomen or pelvis), or other vital organs (e.g. the spleen, heart, aorta).
  Lesions which will be surgically resected regardless of the biopsy result. This applies to many solitary lung and kidney masses.

We have always been concerned with the radiation dose to our patients from various imaging studies, as all of us know CT is a high dose examination. Dose in CT is measured by the effective dose, i.e. dose received by critical organs.

The majority of dose in CT scanning is delivered to the thin volume of tissue (1-10 mm) exposed to the primary beam. Tissues outside this will also receive some dose from scatter radiation.

Radiation dose from CT procedures varies from patient. A particular radiation dose will depend on the size of the body part examined, the type of procedure, and the type of CT equipment and its operation. Typical values cited for radiation dose should be considered as estimates that cannot be precisely associated with any individual patient, examination, or type of CT system. The actual dose from a procedure could be two or three times larger or smaller than the estimates. Facilities performing "screening" procedures may adjust the radiation dose used to levels less (by factors such as 1/2 to 1/5 for so called "low doses CT scans) than those typically used for diagnostic CT procedures.

The quantity most relevant for assessing the risk of cancer detriment from a CT procedures is the effective dose. Effective dose is evaluated in units of millisieverts (abbreviated mSv; 1 mSv = 1 mGv in the case of X-rays). Using the concept of effective dose allows comparison of the risk estimates associated with partial or whole-body radiation exposures. This quantity also incorporates the different rdiation sensitivities of the various organs in the body. Estimates of the effective dose from a diagnostic CT procedure can vary by a factor of 10 or more depending on the type of CT procedure patient size and the CT system and its operating technique. A list of representative diagnostic procedures and associated doses are given in Table 8.1 that is from a report of the European commission.

Table 8.1: Radiation dose comparison			
Diagnostic procedure	Typical effective dose (mSv)[1]	Number of chest X-rays (PA film) for equivalent effective dose[2]	Time period for equivalent effective dose from natural background radiation[3]
Chest X-ray (PA film)	0.02	1	2.4 days
Skull X-ray	0.07	4	8.5 days
Lumbar spine	1.3	65	158 days
IV urogram	2.5	125	304 days
Upper GI exam	3.0	150	1.0 year
Barium enema	7.0	350	2.3 years
CT head	2.0	100	243 days
CT abdomen	10.0	500	3.3 years

The primary dose comes from the acquisition of data for slice recon. Scout scans have a lower radiation dose than their conventional counterparts.

FACTORS AFFECTING RADIATION DOSE
- Scanner generation.
- Rotation angle—360° produce more dose.
- Filtration—decreases the patient dose from removal of low energy X-rays.
- Detector efficiency.

• The patient is observed either in the department or in a short-stay nursing unit for 2 to 4 hours, and then sent home. If there are no complications admission to the hospital is seldom required.

BIOPSY SCAN

Biopsy Scan 1

Function

The biopsy Rx feature allows you to easily repeat the scan location during the biopsy procedures. Example given below is from a CT/E scanner from Ge.

Biopsy Rx Prescription

1. Biopsy Rx can be accessed through the (Biopsy Rx) icon on the righ side of axial/helical prescription screen.
2. The following screen appears upon the selection of (biopsy Rx).

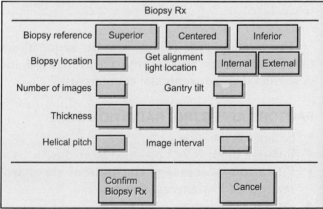

Fig. 6.4: Schematic representation of planning biopsy

Biopsy Scan 2

1. In order to determine the reference centering in a biopsy scan, select (superior), (centered) or (inferior) at biopsy reference field.
   - Superior means scanning from the landmark toward patient's head
   - Centered means scanning around the landmark.
   - Inferior means scanning from the landmark toward patient's feet
2. When the internal light is used, select (internal) or when the external light is used select (external) at Get Alignment Light Location Field.
3. Enter the following parameters:
   - Number of images
   - Gantry tilt
   - Thickness
   - Helical pitch
   - Image interval
4. Click on the (confirm biopsy Rx) button.
5. Press (move to scan) button when it lights up. Then, press (start scan) to start the biopsy scans.

NATIONAL COUNCIL ON RADIATION PROTECTION (NCRP) AND MEASUREMENTS

Occupational Dose Limits

- *50 mSv (5 rem)*—annual effective dose limit
  and
- *10 mSv (1 rem) × age (y)*—cumulative effective dose limit
- *150 mSv (15 rem)*—annual equivalent dose limit to lens of eye
- *500 mSv (50 rem)*—annual equivalent dose limit to skin, hands, and feet

Public Dose Limits

- *1 mSv (0.1 rem)*—annual effective dose limit for continuous exposure
- *5 mSv (0.5 rem)*—annual effective dose limit for infrequent exposure
- *50 mSv (5 rem)*—annual effective dose limit to lens of eye, skin, and extremities

Embryo Fetus

- *0.5 mSv (0.05-50 m rem)*—equivalent dose limit in a month once pregnancy is known..

ESTIMATED RADIATION RISKS POTENTIALLY ASSOCIATED WITH FULL-BODY CT SCREENING

Full-body CT screening of healthy adults is intended to be an early detection device for a variety of diseases including lung cancer, coronary artery disease, and colon cancer.

While the potential benefits and risk have been debated in terms of disease detection vs. false positives, less attention has been paid to the potential radiation risks associated with full-body CT scanning. The radiation issue is pertinent because CT scans by their nature result in much larger organ doses compared with conventional single-film X-rays.

Typical doses from a single full-body scan are about 9 mGy to the lung, 8 mGy to the digestive organs, and 6 mGy to the bone marrow. The effective dose, which is a weighted average of doses to all organs, is about 7 mSv.

In Utero Exposure

Whenever a patient with clinical suspicion of pregnancy needs a scan the potential benefits and risks have to be weighed before a decicion is made for scanning. Following precautions can be taken if the need is very great: (1) shielding of abdomen if the study permits, (2) no of slices can be reduced to a minimum.

Report 54 of the NCRP (National Council for Radiation Protection) is particularly useful for calculating fetal dose. These data include dose received from both direct and indirect exposures.

NCRP reports state that the risk for pregnancy is less at 5 rad (50 mGy) or less when compared to other risks of pregnancy. The risk for malformation is substantially increased at doses above 15 rad (150 mGy).

CT contrast agents, sometimes referred to as "dyes" are used to highlight specific areas so that the organs, blood vessels, or tissues are more visible. By increasing the visibility of all surfaces of the organ or tissue being studied, they can help the radiologist determine the presence and extent of disease or injury.

Contrast agents are available in several different forms, but in general a CT contrast agent is a pharmaceutical substance. Some of the more common contrast agents used are:

- Iodine
- Barium
- Barium sulfate
- Gastrografin

Contrast agents for CT examinations are administered in four different ways:

- Intravenous injection
- Oral administration
- Rectal administration
- Inhalation—This is a relatively uncommon procedure in which xenon gas is inhaled for a highly specialized form of lung or brain imaging. The technique, xenon CT, is only available at a small number of locations worldwide and is used only for rare cases.

INTRAVENOUS CONTRAST

Intravenous contrast is used to highlight blood vessels and to enhance the structure of organs like the brain, spine, liver, and kidney. The contrast agent (usually an iodine compound) is clear, with a water-like consistency. Typically the contrast is contained in a special injector, which injects the contrast through a small needle taped in place (usually on the back of the hand) during a specific period in the CT exam.

Once the contrast is injected into the bloodstream, it circulates throughout the body. The CT's X-ray beam is weakened as it passes through the blood vessels and organs that have "taken up" the contrast. These structures are enhanced by this process and show up as white areas on the CT images. When the test is finished, the kidneys and liver quickly eliminate the contrast from the body.

Iodinated Contrast Agents

Is Iodine a Safe Contrast Agent?

Iodine is considered to be a safe contrast agent. It has been used for many years without serious side effects. Because iodine contrast increases the visibility of target tissues on the images, the benefits are considered to outweigh the risks. The most common side effect of iodine is a warm or "flushed" sensation during the actual injection of the iodine, followed sometimes by a metallic taste in the mouth that usually lasts for less than a minute. No treatment is necessary for this sensation, if experienced.

Another mild reaction is itching over various parts of the body. This reaction lasts from several minutes to a few hours after the injection. When this reaction occurs, medication is usually administered to counteract the itching.

More serious allergic reactions, while uncommon, include difficulty breathing and swelling of the throat

The complex nature of processes involves multiple imaging modalities. Requires an interdisciplinary team of medical and paramedical personnel and techno-logists.

In case of computed tomography, it is the CT technologist who performs the computed tomography examination that creates the images needed for diagnosis. Computed tomography technologists need to integrate scientific knowledge and technical skills with effective patient interaction to provide quality patient care and useful diagnostic information for the radiologist.

NEEDS OF A GOOD COMPUTED TOMOGRAPHY TECHNOLOGIST

The computed tomography technologist must demon-strate an understanding of human cross-sectional anatomy, and medical terminology.

Computed tomography technologists must maintain a high degree of accuracy in positioning and exposure technique. He or she must maintain knowledge about radiation protection and safety.

Computed tomography technologists prepare for and assist the radiologist in the completion of compu-ted tomography examinations including a range of tissue biopsies and fluid drainages. They should supervise or be able to administer contrast media and medications.

Computed tomography technologists are the primary liaison between patients and radiologists and other members of the support team. They must remain sensitive to the physical and emotional needs of the patient through good communication, patient assessment, patient monitoring and patient care skills.

The practice standards define the practice and establish general criteria to determine compliance. They include desired and achievable levels of performance against which actual performance can be measured.

COMPUTED TOMOGRAPHY CLINICAL PERFORMANCE STANDARDS: SUMMARY

Standard one—Assessment: Collect pertinent data about the patient and the procedure.

Standard two—Analysis/Determination: Analyzes the information obtained plan for completing the scan.

Standard three—Patient Education: Provide information about the procedure to the patient.

Standard four—Implementation: Implements the scan and Archives images to data storage devices according to established guidelines.
1. Performs venipuncture,
2. Administers contrast agents according to established guidelines.
3. Monitors the patient for reactions to contrast agent.
4. Uses appropriate radiation safety devices.
5. Monitors the patient's physical condition during the procedure.
6. Applies appropriate patient immobilization devices when necessary.
7. Completes routine camera operations—formats, ensures an adequate film supply for the procedure and verifies image location.

The preparation for rectal contrast is similar to oral contrast, in that the patient should be fasting for several hours before the test. In addition, the patient will be required to use a Fleets Enema to cleanse the colon; it is usually used the night before the examination.

Is Rectal Contrast Safe?

Rectal contrast is considered to be safe and passes through the gastrointestinal tract uneventfully. Minor and temporary side effects, such as constipation, can occur.

Guidelines for IV Contrast Agent Reactions

Q. Radiographic contrast media adverse reactions?
Iodinated contrast media is routinely administered for many radiological procedures like CT, IVP or angiography. Due to the higher absorption of X-ray beams by the iodinated contrast, both normal and abnormal structures are better seen. However, because of the risks of adverse reaction to contrast administration in some patients, judicious use of these agents is required. The following are frequently asked questions about contrast media and contrast reactions.

Q. How frequently do allergic contrast reactions occur?
It is estimated that the overall frequency of adverse reactions is 5 to 10 percent. Most of these are very mild and may consist of only a few hives. However, in one of every 1,000 to 2,000 examinations, a moderate or severe reaction can occur. The risk of death from a

contrast agent is estimated to be 0.3 to 2.6 per 100,000 uses (comparable in magnitude to the risk of death from receiving a dose of penicillin).

Q. What types of allergic contrast reactions are seen?
Contrast reactions are classified as mild, moderate, or severe. Mild reactions include mild nausea and vomiting, mild urticaria and pruritus, and mild diaphoresis. Moderate reactions would include more severe presentations of the above symptoms, facial and laryngeal edema or mild bronchospasm. Severe reactions may include hypotensive shock, cardiac or respiratory arrest, pulmonary edema, loss of consciousness, convulsions, and severe laryngeal or bronchial spasm.

Q. How are these contrast reactions treated?
All contrast examinations are performed in the presence of a physician, usually a radiologist, the technician must be ready to initiate treatment of any reaction (Keep a guidelines for the treatment of these reactions in the CT gantry room). Most reactions are mild and require no treatment; outpatients are usually observed for 30 minutes for worsening of symptoms. In most cases, these mild symptoms are self-limiting and will resolve within this time with minimal or no treatment.

Q. What can be done if a patient with a history of contrast reaction needs another contrast exam?
This depends on the nature and severity of the prior reaction. If the prior reaction was mild, selection of a low-osmolar contrast agent ("non-ionic") and/or pretreatment with 25 to 50 mg of diphenhydramine

Date	Contrast scale			High contrast spatial	Slice thick-ness	Align Y/N	Low contrast resolution			Noise	
		Mean CT #	STD. DEV					Mean CT #		Mean CT #	STD DEV
								Top	Bottom		
	Plexiglas			1.6mm							
	Water			1.3mm			Water				
	Difference		X	1.0mm			Membrane				
				0.8mm			Difference				
							Holes				
	Plexiglas			1.6mm							
	Water			1.3mm			Water				
	Difference		X	1.0mm			Membrane				
				0.8mm			Difference				
							Holes				
	Plexiglas			1.6mm							
	Water			1.3mm			Water				
	Difference		X	1.0mm			Membrane				
				0.8mm			Difference				
							Holes				
	Plexiglas			1.6mm							
	Water			1.3mm			Water				
	Difference		X	1.0mm			Membrane				
				0.8mm			Difference				
							Holes				

Fig. 9.1: Quality assurance DATA form

Radiation Dose

- Factors affecting patient dose
- Dose measurement
- Typical dose values
- Radiation protection.

Quality Check-up

In order to maintain consistent image quality users must establish and actively maintain

- A quality assurance programme
- Quaup phantom
  - High contrast resolution
  - Contrast scale
  - Slice thickness
  - Positioning localizer accuracy
  - Low contrast detectability
  - Noise and uniformity.

PROTOCOLS TO BE KNOWN

Head

- Brain routine
- Brain-axial and coronal
- Posterior fossa
- Trauma
- Circle of Willis
- Pituitary gland—axial and coronal
- Orbits—axial and coronal
- Facial bones—axial and coronal
- Sinuses—axial and coronal
- Internal auditory canals
- Temporomandibular joints—axial and coronal

Neck

- Neck—Routine
- Carotid arteries
- Nasopharynx
- Oral cavity
- Thyroid
- Glottis

Chest

- Chest—Routine
- Hilum
- Aortic dissection
- Aortic aneurysm
- Pulmonary embolism
- High resolution lung

Abdomen and Pelvis

- Abdomen—Routine
- Abdomen—Trauma
- Abdomen and pelvis—Routine
- Aortic Aneurysm
- Liver—Triphase
- Adrenals
- Pancreas—Uniphase
- Kidneys—Routine
- Kidneys—Stone search
- Kidneys—Biphase
- Kidneys—Triphase
- Pelvis—Routine
- Pelvis—Biphase
- Pelvis—Trauma

- Endometrium/Cervix
- Ovary

Spine

- Cervical—Routine
- Cervical—Trauma
- Thoracic—Routine
- Lumbar—Routine
- Lumbar—Disks

Extremities

- Shoulder
- Elbow
- Wrist
- Hip
- Knee
- Ankle
- Calcaneus

Interventional

- CT guided biopsy

CT SECTIONAL ANATOMY

Head

- Brain
- Orbits
- Sinuses
- Temporal bones
- Maxillofacial bones
- Posterior fossa

- TM joints
- Circle of Willis

Neck

- Nasopharynx
- Esophagus
- Larynx
- Musculature
- Vasculature

Spine

- Cervical
- Thoracic
- Lumbar
- Sacrum

Chest

- Mediastinum
- Heart
- Lung
- Pleural space
- Vasculature

Abdomen

- Liver and gallbladder
- GI tract
- Pancreas
- Spleen
- Adrenals
- Kidneys

- Retroperitoneal space
- Vasculature

Pelvis

- Ureters
- Urinary bladder
- Uterus
- Ovaries
- Prostate
- Vasculature

Musculoskeletal

- Upper extremity
- Lower extremity
- Pelvis
- Hips
- Vasculature

STEP BY STEP GUIDE TO A TYPICAL CT EXAMINATION

Request Form

- Check form is fully completed and signed.
- Check pregnancy question if required.
- Check examination request correlates to clinical history.
- Register on computer.
- Take special care with details from, elderly, handicapped, deaf, blind, very young, individuals with poor English etc.
- Review any previous reports and or films.

Request Form + Patient

- Confirm details of patient and examination.
- Check details of any special projection asked.
- Identity, use a positive ID check, use DOB and or address.
- Previous examinations.
- Check and have patient sign for pregnancy risk if appropriate.

Escort Patient to Changing Cubicles

- Give changing instruction relevant to examination.
- Use starch free examination gown and dressing gown.
- Ensure patient's modesty is protected and they are warm enough.
- Instruct patients in the removal of artifacts relevant to the examination, i.e. jewellery and prostheses.

****** **Whilst Patient is Changing** ******

Pre-examination Preparation

*** Collect patient and escort to examination room***

The Examination

- Greet patient and make positive identity check. State your name and grade.
- Check request details match patients' symptoms , i.e. right/left limbs.
  - Inform patient of basic procedure.
  - Position patient.
  - Position gonad protect if required.

- Finalise exposure.
- Rehearse any breathing/moving procedures.
- Instruct patient and visually check them in respiratory manoeuvres or required movements.
- Visually check all round to ensure it is safe to make exposure.
- Expose
- Inform patient to relax and breath normally
- Remove cassette to a safe place
- Proceed with the next position etc.
- When finished escort patient to waiting cubicle and instruct to wait and or to redress if required.
- Mark name on films and process.
- Complete documentation on request form and in computer.

Assessing the CT Film

- Place the radiograph correctly on the viewing box.
- Check, identification, name, date, hospital, registration number.
- Check anatomical marker/legend correct R/L and AP/PA area under examination, limits of examination.

Departure of the Patient

- Inform patient examination is completed.
- Return any jewellery or artifacts removed.
- Inform patient that any dietary preparations are finished and any side/after effects of any drugs or medication e.g. white stools after Barium examinations.

Chapter 10

Computed Tomography Glossary

Artifact (structured noise): The appearance in the CT image of details not present in the scanned object. The main components of structured noise are due to a form of **partial volume effect** and to **beam hardening**. Both effects usually result in streaking artifacts, which are observed in regions of high contrast when there is a sharp discontinuity in object density, such as at air-tissue, air-bone and metal-tissue boundaries. Streaking will also arise from mechanical misalignment within the scanner and, in clinical practice, from patient motion and the use of high-density contrast media.

Attenuation: Reduction of the radiation **intensity**, upon passage through matter, resulting from all types of interaction.

Back projection: Mathematical procedure for the reconstruction of the CT image, based on the smearing of the individual **rays** within a view (projection) back along the direction in which they were measured. Spatial filtration (**convolution**) of the **raw data** is necessary before back projection in order to reduce **artifacts**.

Beam hardening: The process of filtration of a polychromatic beam by the preferential absorption of lower energy photons in tissue, with a subsequent increase in effective energy. The associated artifacts are of particular significance in **quantitative computed tomography (QCT)**.

Calibration of a CT scanner: Correction procedures used to take account of variations in beam intensity or **detector** efficiency in order to achieve homogeneity within the field of view and accuracy of **CT number**. Calibration procedures include scanning air or an appropriate **test phantom**.

Collimation: Geometrical limitation of the extent of the radiation beam in the z-direction.

Computed tomography dose index (CTDI): Integral along a line parallel to the axis of rotation (z) of the **dose profile** (D(z)), measured free-in-air or in a **CT dosimetry phantom** for a single slice, divided by the **nominal slice thickness** (T):

$$CTDI = \frac{1}{T} \int_{-00}^{+00} D(z)dz \qquad \text{(mGy)}$$

In practice, it is convenient to use a pencil ionisation chamber with an active length of 100 mm so as to provide a measurement of $CTDI_{100}$ (mGy to air).

Computed tomography number (CT number): Number used to represent the mean X-ray attenuation associated with each elemental area of the CT image. Numbers are normally expressed in terms of **Hounsfield unit (HU)**. Measured values of **attenuation** are transformed into **CT numbers** using the international Hounsfield scale:

$$CT\ number = \frac{\mu_{material} - \mu_{water}}{\mu_{water}} 1000 \qquad \text{(HU)}$$

Where μ is the effective **linear attenuation coefficient** for the X-ray beam. The CT number scale is defined so that water has a value of 0 HU and air a value of -1000 HU.

Contrast: In relation to the radiation emerging from an irradiated object, if the photon fluence at some reference point is $\emptyset_0$, and at an adjacent point is $\emptyset_1$, the contrast can be defined as $(\emptyset_1 - \emptyset_0) / \emptyset_0$. Contrast can also be expressed in terms of energy fluence or exposure.

Contrast enhancement: Administration of intravenous or intra-arterial contrast increase the visibility of low contrast structures due to increased density of vessels and organs/tissue containing contrast media.

Contrast resolution: See **low contrast resolution**.

Convolution: The mathematical process by which **raw data** undergo spatial filtration prior to **back projection**.

Couch increment: Distance by which position of patient couch (table) is changed between individual slices in serial scanning or the distance the couch position is changed during one 360° rotation of the tube during helical scanning.

CT dosimetry phantoms: Cylinders of **polymethyl-methacrylate (PMMA)** used for standard measure-ments of dose in CT, having a diameter of 16 cm (head phantom) or 32 cm (body phantom) and a length of at least 14 cm. The phantoms are constructed with removable inserts parallel to the axis to allow the positioning of a dosimeter at the centre and 1 cm from the outer surface (periphery).

CT number: Abbreviation for **computed tomography number**.

CTDI: Abbreviation for **computed tomography dose index**.

CTDI$_{air}$: Value of **CTDI** determined free-in-air.

CTDI$_w$: See **weighted CTDI**.

Detector: A single element of a **detector array**, which produces an electrical or light signal in response to stimulation by X-rays.

Detector array: The entire assembly of **detectors**, including their interspace material, arranged along an arc or circumference (depending on scanner technology) of a circle centred on the axis of rotation.

Detector efficiency: For each **detector** contained in a **detector array**, the ratio between the number of pulses recorded and the number of X-ray photons incident on the detector.

Detector width: In a **detector array**, the distance between the two opposite faces of any single **detector**.

Diagnostic reference level: Advisory dose levels set by professional bodies to prompt local reviews of practice if consistently exceeded.

Display matrix: The array of rows and columns of **pixels** in the displayed image, typically between 512 × 512 and 1024 × 1024. It may be equal to or larger than the size of the **reconstruction matrix** due to **interpolation** procedures.

Dose descriptor: Measurable parameter, such as $CTDI_{air}$, $CTDI_w$ or **DLP**, from which the **effective dose** or the organ dose delivered to a patient in a CT examination can be estimated, or the performances of different CT scanners can be compared.

Dose-length product (DLP): Dose descriptor used as an indicator of overall exposure for a complete CT examination in order to allow comparison of performance against a reference dose value set for the purpose of promoting optimisation of patient protection.

$$DLP = \sum_i CTDI_w \cdot T \cdot N \qquad \text{(mGy cm)}$$

Where i represents each scan sequence forming part of an examination, and $CTDI_w$ is the **weighted CTDI** for each of the N slices of thickness T (cm) in the sequence.

Dose profile: Representation of the dose as a function of position along a line perpendicular to the tomographic plane.

Dosimetry phantom: See **CT dosimetry phantom**.

Dynamic scanning: A method of obtaining CT scans in rapid sequence so as, for example, to follow the passage of contrast material through vessels or tissue, or to decrease examination time.

Effective dose: Risk-related quantity used as indicator of overall patient dose. It is defined by the International Commission on Radiological Protection (ICRP) in Publication 60 (1991) as the sum of the weighted absorbed doses in all tissues and organs of the body:

$$E = \sum_{T,R} w_R \cdot w_T \cdot D_T \qquad (mSv)$$

where D_T is the absorbed dose (mGy) in tissue T due to radiation R, w_R is the weighting factor for radiation R and w_T is the weighting factor for tissue T. For X-rays, w_R is equal to unity.

Exposure factors: The settings of X-ray tube voltage (kV), tube current (mA) and **exposure time** (s).

Exposure time: Duration of emission of radiation by the X-ray tube (seconds) for an individual slice in axial scanning or total acquisition time for helical scanning.

Field of view (FOV): The maximum diameter of the reconstructed image.

Filter: Mathematical procedure used for the **convolution** of the attenuation profiles and the consequent reconstruction of the CT image.

Focal spot: The effective area on the X-ray tube anode from which X-rays are emitted. The size of the focal spot has influence on **spatial resolution**.

Full width at half maximum (FWHM): Interval parallel to the abscissa between the points on a curve with the value of one-half of the maximum of the symmetrical curve.

Gantry: Scanner structure containing the X-ray tube, collimators and the **detector array**.

Gantry aperture: Diameter of the physical opening of the **gantry** through which the patient is moved for the examination.

Gantry tilt: The angle between the vertical plane, and the plane containing the X-ray fan beam and the **detector array**.

Helical CT: A particular technique of scanning in which there is continuous rotation of the X-ray tube coupled with continuous linear translation of the patient through the **gantry aperture** in order to achieve volumetric data acquisition. Also known as **spiral** or **volume CT**.

High contrast resolution: See **spatial resolution**.

HU (Hounsfield unit): See **CT number**.

Imaging volume: See **volume of investigation**.

Intensity: The quantity of radiation energy flowing through unit area in unit time.

Interpolation: A mathematical method of averaging or smoothing images that are being displayed on a larger number of **pixels** than that for which they were originally reconstructed.

Inter-slice distance: The distance between the adjacent nominal margins of consecutive slices in serial CT scanning. It is dependent upon the couch increment between slices.

Linearity: In CT, the extent to which the **CT number** of a given material is exactly proportional to its density (in HU unit).

Linear attenuation coefficient: The fractional reduction in intensity per unit thickness of material as an X-ray beam passes through an absorber. For a polychromatic beam, the effective linear attenuation coefficient depends on the effective energy of the beam, and the density and atomic number (composition) of the material.

Kernel: See **filter**.

Low contrast resolution: A measure of the ability to discriminate between structures with slightly differing attenuation properties (**CT number**). It depends on the stochastic **noise** and is usually expressed as the minimum detectable size of detail discernable in the image, for a fixed percentage difference in contrast relative to the adjacent background.

Monte Carlo Technique: A technique for obtaining an approximate solution to certain mathematical and physical problems, characteristically involving the replacement of a probability distribution by sample values, usually performed using a computer.

Multiple scan average dose (MSAD): The MSAD is the average dose across the central slice from a series of N slices (each of thickness T) when there is a constant increment I between successive slices:

$$MSAD = \frac{1}{I} \int_{-\frac{1}{2}}^{+\frac{1}{2}} D_{N,I}(z)\,dz \qquad (mGy)$$

Where $D_{N,I}(z)$ is the multiple scan dose profile along a line parallel to the axis of rotation (z). For a sufficient number of slices such that the first and the last in the series do not contribute any significant dose over the width of the central slice:

$$MSAD = \frac{T}{I}\, CTDI \qquad (mGy)$$

Noise: Noise is the point-to-point variation in image density that does not contain useful information. The magnitude of noise is indicated by the percentage standard deviation of the **CT numbers** within a **region of interest** in the image of a uniform substance (generally water), relative to the difference in CT numbers between water and air.

Nominal (tomographic) slice thickness: The **slice thickness** selected and indicated at the control panel of the CT scanner.

Number of measurements: The total number of attenuation values measured during the acquisition of the **raw data** for a single slice.

Packing factor: In relation to dosimetry for serial CT, the packing factor (p) is used to spread the radiation density evenly over the **volume of investigation** when the slices are not contiguous. For a series of N slices, each of thickness T, and with a **couch increment** I such that the total scan length is L:

$$CT\ pitch\ factor = \frac{\Delta d}{N \times T}$$

P = 1 for contiguous slices
p > 1 for overlapping slices
p < 1 for gaps between slices.

Partial volume effect: The inaccuracy in **CT number** caused by the presence of a structure within only part of a **slice**. Such effects become less important as the **slice thickness** is reduced.

Pitch factor: In relation to helical CT, ratio of the patient couch travel in horizontal direction per rotation of the X-ray tube divided by the product of the number of tomographic sections produced by a single rotation of the X-ray tube N times the **nominal tomographic slice thickness** T:

$$CT \text{ pitch factor } = \frac{\Delta d}{N \times T}$$

Where:

Delta d *is the patient couch travel in horizontal direction*

N is the number of tomographic sections produced by a single rotation of the X-ray tube

T is the **nominal tomographic slice thickness**.

Pixel: Individual square picture element of a digital image display, being the two-dimensional representation in **HU** of a **voxel** within the scanned slice. Pixel size is determined by the diameter of the **field of view** and the number of elements in the **display matrix**.

Polymethylmethacrylate (PMMA): Polymethylmethacrylate, a polymer plastic commercially available for example as Perspex or Lucite.

Profile of CT numbers: Representation of the **CT numbers** of the **pixels** along a specified direction in a CT image.

Quantitative computed tomography (QCT): The use of CT images and the corresponding **CT numbers** for quantitative characterization of organs or tissues. QCT is most-widely used in relation to the determination of bone mineral content and treatment planning in radiotherapy.

Radiographic exposure: Product of tube current and exposure time.

Raw data: The values of X-ray **detector** response from all views and **rays** within a scan. These data are convolved with the **convolution** filter and undergo **back projection** to produce a CT image.

Ray: The narrow beam of X-rays from the tube **focal spot** to a single **detector** within a **detector array**, giving rise to a detector reading. Each view or projection is composed of numerous rays.

Reconstruction algorithm: Mathematical procedure used to convert **raw data** into an image. Different algorithms are used to emphasize, enhance, or improve certain aspects of the data.

Reconstruction matrix: The array of rows and columns of **pixels** in the reconstructed image.

Region of interest (ROI): Localised part of an image defined by the operator which is of particular interest at a given time.

Ring artifacts: Circular **artifacts**, usually found in third-generation scanners, caused by faulty calibration or a defect in detector function.

Scanning: The process of recording X-ray attenuation data through a slice of an object, from which images are reconstructed.

Scan projection radiograph (SPR): Generic name for the digital image obtained by linearly translating the patient through the **gantry aperture** during an X-ray exposure while the X-ray tube remains stationary. The SPR has a similar appearance to a plain radiograph and is used primarily for localizing the required region of scanning. Synonymous terms include radiographic mode and localizer image, together with the proprietary names Pilot scan, Scanogram, Scanoscope, Scoutview, Surview and Topogram.

Scan time: The time interval between the beginning and the end of the acquisition of **attenuation** data for a single exposure. For some CT scanners, this may be longer than the **exposure time** due to the pulsing of X-ray emission.

Scattered radiation: Secondary radiation belonging to the same radiation type as the original radiation, produced in the interaction of the original radiation with a material medium. The interaction can be characterized by a reduction in radiation energy and/or by a change in the direction of the radiation.

Sensitivity profile: Relative response of a system for CT as a function of position along a line perpendicular to the tomographic plane.

Signal to noise ratio: The ratio of the strength of the signal for information content in the image to the noise level (the standard deviation of the signal).

Slice: Tomographic section (defined by position and thickness) of a **test phantom** or patient under investigation during a single CT exposure in serial scanning.

Slice thickness: Effective thickness of the tomographic section, as measured by the **full width at half maximum** of the **sensitivity profile** in the centre of the scan field.

Spatial resolution (or high contrast resolution): The ability to resolve different objects in the displayed CT image, when the difference in **attenuation** between the objects and the background is large compared to **noise**; normally a difference corresponding to at least one hundred **HU** is considered adequate.

Spiral CT: See **helical CT**.

Stability: The maintenance over time of constancy of **CT numbers** and **uniformity**.

Standard examination: Outline of scanning procedure for a particular clinical indication that is generally accepted as being able to provide adequate clinical information in most of the patients examined.

Test phantom: Object of particular shape, size and structure (including standardised representations of human form), used for the purposes of calibration and evaluation of performance of CT scanners.

Uniformity: Consistency of the **CT numbers** in the image of a homogeneous material across the scan field.

Volume CT: See **helical CT**.

Volume of investigation (imaging volume): Entire volume of the region under investigation by scanning.

Voxel: Elementary volume element (expressed in units of mm^3) within the scanned slice of the object, with which **CT numbers** are associated.

Weighted CTDI ($CTDI_w$): An estimate of the average dose over a single slice in a **CT dosimetry phantom** that is used to allow comparison of performance against a reference dose value set for the purpose of promoting optimisation of patient protection.

$$CTDI_w = (1/3 \, CTDI_{100,c} + 2/3 \, CTDI_{100,p}) \quad \text{(mGy)}$$

Where $CTDI_{100,c \text{ or } p}$ refer to measurements of $CTDI_{100}$ at the centre (c) or periphery (p) of the head or body phantom for the settings used in clinical practice.

Window level: The central value of the window (in **HU**) used for the display of the reconstructed image on the image monitor of the CT scanner.

Window setting: The setting of the **window level** and the **window width**, selected for optimization of the grey scale levels in the displayed CT-image.

Window width: The range of **CT numbers** within which the entire grey scale is displayed on the image monitor of the CT scanner.

Index